Seizure Solutions: A Practical Guide to Managing Epilepsy

N.B. Singh

DEDICATION

To Nature,

I dedicate this book to you, the source of all life. You are my inspiration, my teacher, and my friend.

Thank you for teaching me about the beauty of the world around me. Thank you for showing me the power of the natural world. Thank you for giving me a sense of peace and tranquillity.

I promise to do my part to protect you and your many wonders. I will teach my children about the importance of conservation and sustainability. I will work to make the world a better place for all living things.

Thank you for everything, Nature.

With love,

N.B Singh

Contents

6   Coping Strategies   53

PREFACE

Living with epilepsy presents unique challenges, not only for the individuals who experience seizures but also for their loved ones and caregivers. "Seizure Solutions" aims to be a comprehensive and practical guide to managing epilepsy, offering insights, strategies, and support for navigating the complexities of this condition.

This book is a result of both personal experiences and extensive research in the field of epilepsy management. It combines medical knowledge with real-life stories, providing a holistic perspective on the challenges and triumphs associated with epilepsy.

Structure of the Book: Each chapter addresses a specific aspect of epilepsy, from understanding different seizure types to coping strategies, medication management, and considerations for various life stages. The content is presented in an accessible manner, making it suitable for individuals living with epilepsy, their families, and healthcare professionals.

Who Can Benefit: Whether you have been recently diagnosed with epilepsy, are a long-time epilepsy warrior, or are a caregiver seeking guidance, "Seizure Solutions" is designed to empower you with knowledge and practical solutions. It serves as a roadmap for creating a tailored approach to managing epilepsy based on individual needs and circumstances.

I invite you to explore the pages of "Seizure Solutions" and embark on a journey towards better understanding, management, and ultimately, a fulfilling life with epilepsy.

N.B. Singh

Chapter 1

Introduction

1.1 Understanding Epilepsy

Epilepsy is a neurological disorder characterized by recurrent seizures, which are abnormal bursts of electrical activity in the brain. These seizures can manifest in various ways, from momentary lapses in awareness to full-body convulsions.

1.1.1 The Basics of Brain Activity

To grasp epilepsy, it's essential to understand the basics of brain function. The brain consists of billions of neurons communicating through electrical signals. Neurons use neurotransmitters to transmit signals across synapses, creating a delicate balance of excitation and inhibition.

1.1.2 Seizure Triggers

Seizures can be triggered by imbalances in neurotransmitters, sudden bursts of abnormal electrical activity, or structural abnormalities in the brain. Identifying and managing these triggers is crucial in epilepsy management.

1.1.3 The Seizure Threshold Equation

A simple model to conceptualize seizure occurrence is the Seizure Threshold Equation:

$$\text{Seizure Threshold} = \text{Excitation} - \text{Inhibition}$$

Understanding this equation helps in appreciating factors influencing seizure occurrence. Both excitatory and inhibitory factors play vital roles.

1.1.4 Medication Mechanisms

Anti-epileptic medications aim to restore the balance by either enhancing inhibition or suppressing excitation. The drug effect can be mathematically represented:

$$\text{Drug Effect} = \text{Inhibition Enhancement} - \text{Excitation Suppression}$$

1.1.5 Ion Channel Dynamics

At a molecular level, seizures involve disruptions in ion channel dynamics. The Hodgkin-Huxley model mathematically describes how ion channels contribute to the generation of electrical impulses in neurons.

$$C_m \frac{dV}{dt} = I_{\text{ion}} + I_{\text{stim}} \tag{1.1}$$

Where C_m is the membrane capacitance, V is the membrane potential, I_{ion} is the ion current, and I_{stim} is the stimulus current.

1.1.6 Chemical Imbalance

The imbalance of neurotransmitters, such as GABA and glutamate, plays a pivotal role in seizure genesis. This chemical equilibrium can be expressed in a simplified form:

$$\text{GABA} - \text{Glutamate} = \text{Seizure Susceptibility}$$

Understanding these mathematical aspects provides a foundation for comprehending epilepsy on both a macroscopic and microscopic level.

1.2 Types of Seizures

Seizures come in various forms, each with unique characteristics. Understanding these types is crucial for effective epilepsy management.

1.2.1 Generalized Seizures

Tonic-Clonic Seizures

This common seizure type involves two distinct phases. The tonic phase is characterized by muscle stiffness, and the clonic phase involves rhythmic jerking movements. The total duration of the seizure is a key factor in assessment.

$$\text{Total Seizure Duration} = \text{Tonic Duration} + \text{Clonic Duration}$$

Absence Seizures

Absence seizures are brief episodes of staring or blankness, often mistaken for daydreaming. They are associated with a sudden loss of awareness and typically last for a few seconds.

$$\text{Frequency of Absence Seizures} = \frac{\text{Number of Absence Seizures}}{\text{Monitoring Time}}$$

1.2.2 Partial (Focal) Seizures

Simple Partial Seizures

These seizures affect a specific part of the brain, leading to localized symptoms. No loss of consciousness occurs. The Jacksonian march can be observed, indicating the progression of symptoms through specific body parts.

$$\text{Jacksonian March} = \text{Sequential Involvement of Body Parts}$$

Complex Partial Seizures

Complex partial seizures involve altered consciousness and can manifest as automatic behaviors. The focus of the seizure is within a specific brain region, often originating from the temporal lobe.

$$\text{Temporal Lobe Activity} = \text{Complex Partial Seizure Susceptibility}$$

1.2.3   Other Seizure Types

Myoclonic Seizures

Myoclonic seizures are characterized by brief, jerking muscle contractions. They can affect a specific muscle group or involve the entire body.

$$\text{Muscle Group Affected} = \text{Myoclonic Seizure Intensity}$$

Atonic Seizures

Atonic seizures, also known as drop attacks, result in a sudden loss of muscle tone. Understanding the duration and frequency of these seizures is crucial for management.

$$\text{Atonic Seizure Frequency} = \frac{\text{Number of Atonic Seizures}}{\text{Observation Period}}$$

In summary, the diverse nature of seizures necessitates a tailored approach to management, considering factors such as seizure type, duration, and frequency.

1.3   Epilepsy Causes and Triggers

Identifying the causes and triggers of epilepsy is crucial for effective management. Let's explore these factors in a concise and practical manner.

1.3.1   Genetic Factors

Genetics plays a significant role in epilepsy. The probability of inheriting epilepsy can be expressed using a simple genetic probability equation:

$$\text{Genetic Probability} = \frac{\text{Number of Affected Family Members}}{\text{Total Family Members}}$$

Understanding family history aids in assessing the genetic component.

1.3.2   Structural Abnormalities

Brain structure abnormalities, such as tumors or lesions, can contribute to epilepsy. The impact of structural abnormalities can be mathematically conceptualized:

$$\text{Structural Abnormality Impact} = \text{Size of Abnormality} \times \text{Proximity to Seizure Focus}$$

1.3.3 Traumatic Brain Injury (TBI)

Head injuries increase the risk of epilepsy. The likelihood of epilepsy post-TBI can be estimated using the following equation:

$$\text{Epilepsy Risk after TBI} = \frac{\text{Number of TBIs}}{\text{Total Number of Individuals}}$$

1.3.4 Infections and Neurological Disorders

Certain infections and neurological disorders can trigger epilepsy. The relationship between these factors can be expressed as:

$$\text{Infection/Neurological Disorder Impact} = \text{Severity of Infection/Disorder} \times \text{Individual Susceptibility}$$

1.3.5 Metabolic and Developmental Factors

Imbalances in metabolic processes and developmental issues can influence epilepsy. The metabolic factor can be quantified as:

$$\text{Metabolic Imbalance Index} = \frac{\text{Metabolic Disturbances}}{\text{Total Metabolic Factors}}$$

1.3.6 Environmental Triggers

External factors, such as exposure to certain chemicals or flashing lights, can trigger seizures. The impact of environmental triggers can be assessed using:

$$\text{Environmental Trigger Sensitivity} = \text{Exposure Intensity} \times \text{Individual Sensitivity}$$

By understanding and quantifying these causes and triggers, individuals and healthcare professionals can develop personalized strategies for epilepsy management.

1.4   Treatment Options

Exploring treatment options for epilepsy involves considering various strategies and their practical implications. Let's delve into these approaches in a concise and memorable manner.

1.4.1   Anti-Seizure Medications

Medication Selection Criteria

Choosing the right medication involves assessing factors such as seizure type, potential side effects, and lifestyle considerations. A decision matrix can aid in selecting the most suitable option:

$$\text{Medication Suitability Index} = \frac{\text{Efficacy} \times \text{Side Effect Tolerance}}{\text{Dosage Frequency}}$$

Dose Adjustment

Adjusting medication doses is a common practice. The dosage adjustment factor can be expressed as:

$$\text{Dosage Adjustment Factor} = \frac{\text{Current Dosage}}{\text{Target Dosage}}$$

1.4.2   Surgical Interventions

Resective Surgery Considerations

For cases where medication is ineffective, resective surgery may be an option. Assessing the potential success of resective surgery involves considering the following equation:

$$\text{Resective Surgery Success Probability} = \frac{\text{Seizure-Free Cases}}{\text{Total Cases Considered}}$$

Vagus Nerve Stimulation (VNS)

VNS is a neuromodulation technique. Its effectiveness can be evaluated using:

$$\text{VNS Effectiveness Index} = \frac{\text{Reduction in Seizure Frequency}}{\text{Device-related Side Effects}}$$

1.4.3 Ketogenic Diet

The ketogenic diet is a non-pharmacological option. Its impact on seizure control can be quantified by:

$$\text{Ketogenic Diet Response Rate} = \frac{\text{Seizure Reduction}}{\text{Adherence Level}}$$

1.4.4 Neurostimulation Devices

Devices like responsive neurostimulation (RNS) monitor brain activity. The effectiveness of RNS can be measured by:

$$\text{RNS Effectiveness} = \frac{\text{Seizure Reduction}}{\text{Incident Triggering Rate}}$$

1.4.5 Complementary Therapies

Acupuncture

The impact of acupuncture on seizure frequency can be assessed through:

$$\text{Acupuncture Success Rate} = \frac{\text{Seizure Reduction}}{\text{Number of Sessions}}$$

Yoga and Mindfulness

The efficacy of yoga and mindfulness interventions can be measured by:

$$\text{Mindfulness Impact} = \frac{\text{Stress Reduction}}{\text{Regular Practice Duration}}$$

Understanding the practical aspects and quantitative measures of these treatment options is vital for informed decision-making in epilepsy management.

1.5 The Importance of Self-Management

Recognizing the significance of self-management in epilepsy is crucial for optimizing overall well-being. Let's explore this concept in a fast and practical manner.

1.5.1 Seizure Diary Impact

Maintaining a seizure diary helps in tracking patterns. The impact of consistent diary use on seizure management can be expressed as:

$$\text{Seizure Diary Adherence} = \frac{\text{Number of Entries}}{\text{Total Days}}$$

1.5.2 Medication Adherence

Consistent medication intake is vital. The Medication Adherence Index provides a measure:

$$\text{Medication Adherence Index} = \frac{\text{Taken Doses}}{\text{Prescribed Doses}}$$

1.5.3 Lifestyle Modifications

Adopting a healthy lifestyle is key. The Lifestyle Improvement Score considers factors like diet, exercise, and stress management:

$$\text{Lifestyle Improvement Score} = \frac{\text{Positive Lifestyle Choices}}{\text{Total Lifestyle Factors}}$$

1.5.4 Sleep Hygiene

Quality sleep contributes to seizure control. The Sleep Quality Equation assesses sleep hygiene:

$$\text{Sleep Quality} = \frac{\text{Hours of Restful Sleep}}{\text{Total Sleep Time}}$$

1.5.5 Stress Management

Effective stress management is vital. The Stress Reduction Factor can quantify the impact:

$$\text{Stress Reduction Factor} = \frac{\text{Reduced Stress Episodes}}{\text{Applied Stress Management Techniques}}$$

1.5.6 Trigger Avoidance

Identifying and avoiding triggers is a proactive approach. The Trigger Avoidance Rate is a measure of success:

$$\text{Trigger Avoidance Rate} = \frac{\text{Avoided Triggers}}{\text{Total Identified Triggers}}$$

1.5.7 Emergency Preparedness

Being prepared for emergencies is empowering. The Emergency Response Efficiency can be gauged by:

$$\text{Emergency Response Efficiency} = \frac{\text{Timely Actions Taken}}{\text{Total Emergency Incidents}}$$

Embracing self-management involves incorporating these practical measures into daily life, ultimately enhancing the ability to navigate and control epilepsy effectively.

1.6 Seeking Professional Help

Knowing when and how to seek professional assistance is pivotal in managing epilepsy. Let's explore this in a fast and practical manner.

1.6.1 Appointment Scheduling Efficiency

Efficiently scheduling appointments is crucial. The Appointment Response Index evaluates the promptness:

$$\text{Appointment Response Index} = \frac{\text{Scheduled Appointments}}{\text{Total Appointment Requests}}$$

1.6.2 Effective Communication

Open communication is key. The Communication Effectiveness Quotient assesses the clarity and understanding:

$$\text{Communication Effectiveness Quotient} = \frac{\text{Clear Interactions}}{\text{Total Communications}}$$

1.6.3 Medication Adjustment Timeliness

Timely adjustments to medication are essential. The Medication Adjustment Timeframe gauges the efficiency:

$$\text{Medication Adjustment Timeframe} = \frac{\text{Timely Adjustments}}{\text{Total Adjustments Needed}}$$

1.6.4 Emergency Response Collaboration

Collaboration during emergencies is vital. The Emergency Response Collaboration Score considers teamwork:

$$\text{Emergency Response Collaboration Score} = \frac{\text{Collaborative Actions}}{\text{Total Emergency Incidents}}$$

1.6.5 Diagnostic Speed

Swift diagnostics aid in effective management. The Diagnostic Speed Index quantifies the efficiency:

$$\text{Diagnostic Speed Index} = \frac{\text{Time to Diagnosis}}{\text{Severity of the Case}}$$

1.6.6 Referral Success

Referrals to specialists contribute to comprehensive care. The Referral Success Rate evaluates the effectiveness:

$$\text{Referral Success Rate} = \frac{\text{Successful Referrals}}{\text{Total Referral Cases}}$$

1.6.7 Continuous Education Impact

Education is an ongoing process. The Continuous Education Impact measures knowledge retention:

$$\text{Continuous Education Impact} = \frac{\text{Applied Knowledge}}{\text{Total Educational Modules}}$$

By proactively engaging with healthcare professionals and optimizing these factors, individuals with epilepsy can enhance the quality of care received and overall health outcomes.

1.7 Living a Full Life with Epilepsy

Embracing a fulfilling life while managing epilepsy involves practical strategies. Let's explore these in a fast and memorable manner.

1.7.1 Social Engagement Equation

Maintaining an active social life is essential. The Social Engagement Equation gauges interaction frequency:

$$\text{Social Engagement Index} = \frac{\text{Social Events Attended}}{\text{Total Invitations Received}}$$

1.7.2 Career Productivity Index

Sustaining a successful career is achievable. The Career Productivity Index quantifies work performance:

$$\text{Career Productivity Index} = \frac{\text{Productive Days}}{\text{Total Workdays}}$$

1.7.3 Adventure and Travel Rating

Exploring the world is possible. The Adventure and Travel Rating assesses the success of travel endeavors:

$$\text{Adventure and Travel Rating} = \frac{\text{Memorable Experiences}}{\text{Total Travel Attempts}}$$

1.7.4 Hobbies and Leisure Satisfaction

Pursuing hobbies enriches life. The Hobbies and Leisure Satisfaction Formula measures fulfillment:

$$\text{Hobbies Satisfaction} = \frac{\text{Enjoyable Hobby Activities}}{\text{Total Hobby Pursuits}}$$

1.7.5 Educational Pursuit Efficiency

Continuous learning is empowering. The Educational Pursuit Efficiency evaluates knowledge acquisition:

$$\text{Educational Pursuit Efficiency} = \frac{\text{Applied Knowledge}}{\text{Total Educational Endeavors}}$$

1.7.6 Emotional Well-being Balance

Balancing emotions is crucial. The Emotional Well-being Index considers mood stability:

$$\text{Emotional Well-being Index} = \frac{\text{Positive Emotional States}}{\text{Total Emotional States Recorded}}$$

1.7.7 Adaptability Quotient

Adaptability is a key trait. The Adaptability Quotient assesses the ability to cope with changes:

$$\text{Adaptability Quotient} = \frac{\text{Successfully Navigated Changes}}{\text{Total Challenging Situations}}$$

By integrating these practical measures into daily life, individuals with epilepsy can lead fulfilling and enriched lives.

Chapter 2

Diagnosis and Testing

2.1 The Diagnostic Process

Navigating the diagnostic process efficiently is vital. Let's explore this in a fast and practical manner.

2.1.1 Seizure Frequency Assessment

Quantifying seizure frequency is a key diagnostic step. The Seizure Frequency Calculation considers the following:

$$\text{Seizure Frequency} = \frac{\text{Number of Seizures}}{\text{Observation Period}}$$

2.1.2 Neurological Examination Score

The neurological exam is crucial for assessment. The Neurological Examination Score evaluates:

$$\text{Neurological Exam Score} = \frac{\text{Normal Responses}}{\text{Total Exam Components}}$$

2.1.3 Diagnostic Imaging Efficiency

Utilizing imaging techniques is common. The Diagnostic Imaging Efficiency Formula quantifies effectiveness:

$$\text{Diagnostic Imaging Efficiency} = \frac{\text{Correctly Identified Abnormalities}}{\text{Total Imaging Tests}}$$

2.1.4 EEG Pattern Recognition

Analyzing EEG patterns aids diagnosis. The EEG Pattern Recognition Index assesses accuracy:

$$\text{EEG Pattern Recognition Index} = \frac{\text{Correct Pattern Identifications}}{\text{Total EEG Analyses}}$$

2.1.5 Blood Test Diagnostic Yield

Blood tests contribute to diagnosis. The Blood Test Diagnostic Yield measures effectiveness:

$$\text{Blood Test Diagnostic Yield} = \frac{\text{Confirmed Diagnoses}}{\text{Total Blood Tests Conducted}}$$

2.1.6 Patient History Relevance

Patient history guides diagnosis. The Patient History Relevance Ratio considers:

$$\text{History Relevance Ratio} = \frac{\text{Relevant Historical Information}}{\text{Total Patient History Components}}$$

2.1.7 Genetic Testing Impact

Genetic testing plays a role. The Genetic Testing Impact Factor quantifies significance:

$$\text{Genetic Testing Impact} = \frac{\text{Informative Genetic Results}}{\text{Total Genetic Tests Conducted}}$$

Efficiently moving through these diagnostic steps aids in a timely and accurate understanding of epilepsy.

2.2 Neurological Examinations

Efficiently conducting neurological examinations is crucial. Let's explore this in a fast and practical manner.

2.2.1 Neurological Exam Scoring

Scoring neurological exams is essential for evaluation. The Neurological Exam Score considers:

$$\text{Neurological Exam Score} = \frac{\text{Normal Responses}}{\text{Total Exam Components}}$$

2.2.2 Reflex Grading Formula

Grading reflex responses provides insights. The Reflex Grading Formula assesses:

$$\text{Reflex Grading} = \frac{\text{Normal Reflexes}}{\text{Total Reflexes Tested}}$$

2.2.3 Sensory Perception Index

Assessing sensory perception aids diagnosis. The Sensory Perception Index considers:

$$\text{Sensory Perception Index} = \frac{\text{Accurate Sensory Responses}}{\text{Total Sensory Tests}}$$

2.2.4 Motor Skills Efficiency

Evaluating motor skills is fundamental. The Motor Skills Efficiency Formula quantifies:

$$\text{Motor Skills Efficiency} = \frac{\text{Precise Motor Responses}}{\text{Total Motor Tasks}}$$

2.2.5 Coordination Assessment

Coordination assessment is vital. The Coordination Success Ratio evaluates:

$$\text{Coordination Success Ratio} = \frac{\text{Coordinated Movements}}{\text{Total Coordination Tasks}}$$

2.2.6 Cranial Nerve Evaluation

Cranial nerve function impacts diagnosis. The Cranial Nerve Evaluation Index measures:

$$\text{Cranial Nerve Evaluation Index} = \frac{\text{Normal Cranial Nerve Functions}}{\text{Total Cranial Nerve Components}}$$

2.2.7   Gait Analysis Efficiency

Analyzing gait provides valuable information. The Gait Analysis Efficiency Formula is expressed as:

$$\text{Gait Analysis Efficiency} = \frac{\text{Steady Gait Instances}}{\text{Total Gait Observations}}$$

Efficiently applying these neurological examination measures enhances the accuracy of epilepsy assessments.

2.3   Diagnostic Tests

Efficiently understanding diagnostic tests is crucial. Let's explore this in a fast and practical manner.

2.3.1   EEG Analysis Speed

Analyzing EEG patterns promptly aids diagnosis. The EEG Analysis Speed Index is calculated as:

$$\text{EEG Analysis Speed Index} = \frac{\text{Cases Analyzed in Time}}{\text{Total EEG Analyses}}$$

2.3.2   MRI Sensitivity

MRI sensitivity is vital for detecting abnormalities. The MRI Sensitivity Formula quantifies this:

$$\text{MRI Sensitivity} = \frac{\text{Correctly Identified Abnormalities}}{\text{Total Abnormalities Present}}$$

2.3.3   Blood Test Specificity

Blood tests contribute to diagnosis. The Blood Test Specificity Ratio is expressed as:

$$\text{Blood Test Specificity Ratio} = \frac{\text{Confirmed Diagnoses}}{\text{Total Blood Tests Conducted}}$$

2.3.4   Genetic Testing Accuracy

Genetic testing provides valuable information. The Genetic Testing Accuracy Index is calculated as:

$$\text{Genetic Testing Accuracy Index} = \frac{\text{Correct Genetic Identifications}}{\text{Total Genetic Tests Conducted}}$$

2.3.5 CSF Analysis Efficiency

Analyzing cerebrospinal fluid (CSF) is critical. The CSF Analysis Efficiency Formula is expressed as:

$$\text{CSF Analysis Efficiency} = \frac{\text{Accurate CSF Analyses}}{\text{Total CSF Tests}}$$

2.3.6 Provocative Seizure Test Success

Provocative seizure tests assist in diagnosis. The Provocative Seizure Test Success Rate is calculated as:

$$\text{Provocative Seizure Test Success Rate} = \frac{\text{Successful Seizure Provocations}}{\text{Total Tests Conducted}}$$

Efficiently applying and interpreting these diagnostic test measures enhances the precision of epilepsy diagnosis.

2.4 Interpreting EEG Results

Quickly interpreting EEG results is crucial. Let's explore this in a fast and practical manner.

2.4.1 Seizure Frequency Assessment

Understanding seizure frequency is key. The Seizure Frequency Calculation considers:

$$\text{Seizure Frequency} = \frac{\text{Number of Seizures}}{\text{Observation Period}}$$

2.4.2 Identifying Focal Points

Identifying focal points is essential for targeted treatment. The Focal Point Localization Index assesses accuracy:

$$\text{Focal Point Localization Index} = \frac{\text{Correctly Identified Focal Points}}{\text{Total Focal Points}}$$

2.4.3   Analyzing Interictal Spikes

Interictal spikes provide diagnostic insights. The Interictal Spike Analysis Score is expressed as:

$$\text{Interictal Spike Analysis Score} = \frac{\text{Correctly Identified Spikes}}{\text{Total Spikes Observed}}$$

2.4.4   Evaluating Background Rhythms

Background rhythms indicate brain activity. The Background Rhythm Evaluation considers:

$$\text{Background Rhythm Evaluation} = \frac{\text{Normal Rhythms Detected}}{\text{Total Background Rhythms}}$$

2.4.5   Quantifying Burst Suppression

Burst suppression patterns reveal abnormalities. The Burst Suppression Quantification Formula is expressed as:

$$\text{Burst Suppression Quantification} = \frac{\text{Correctly Quantified Bursts}}{\text{Total Burst Suppression Instances}}$$

2.4.6   Assessing ictal Patterns

Identifying ictal patterns is crucial. The Ictal Pattern Recognition Index assesses effectiveness:

$$\text{Ictal Pattern Recognition Index} = \frac{\text{Accurate Identification of Ictal Patterns}}{\text{Total Ictal Patterns Observed}}$$

Efficiently interpreting EEG results using these measures enhances diagnostic precision in epilepsy assessment.

2.5   Imaging Techniques

Mastering imaging techniques is vital. Let's explore this in a fast and practical manner.

2.5.1   MRI Sensitivity

MRI sensitivity is crucial for detecting abnormalities. The MRI Sensitivity Formula quantifies this:

$$\text{MRI Sensitivity} = \frac{\text{Correctly Identified Abnormalities}}{\text{Total Abnormalities Present}}$$

2.5.2 CT Scan Specificity

CT scans contribute valuable information. The CT Scan Specificity Ratio is expressed as:

$$\text{CT Scan Specificity Ratio} = \frac{\text{Confirmed Diagnoses}}{\text{Total CT Scans Conducted}}$$

2.5.3 PET Scan Precision

PET scans provide functional insights. The PET Scan Precision Index is calculated as:

$$\text{PET Scan Precision Index} = \frac{\text{Accurate Functional Information}}{\text{Total PET Scans Conducted}}$$

2.5.4 SPECT Imaging Accuracy

SPECT imaging aids in diagnosis. The SPECT Imaging Accuracy Score is expressed as:

$$\text{SPECT Imaging Accuracy Score} = \frac{\text{Correctly Identified Regions}}{\text{Total SPECT Images Analyzed}}$$

2.5.5 Functional MRI Effectiveness

Functional MRI measures brain activity. The Functional MRI Effectiveness Formula is calculated as:

$$\text{Functional MRI Effectiveness} = \frac{\text{Accurate Activation Detection}}{\text{Total Functional MRI Scans}}$$

2.5.6 Angiogram Efficiency

Angiograms assess blood vessels. The Angiogram Efficiency Index quantifies effectiveness:

$$\text{Angiogram Efficiency Index} = \frac{\text{Clear Vessel Visualization}}{\text{Total Angiograms Conducted}}$$

Efficiently mastering these imaging techniques enhances the diagnostic capabilities in epilepsy assessments.

2.6 Genetic Testing

Understanding genetic testing is vital. Let's explore this in a fast and practical manner.

2.6.1 Genetic Probability

Assessing genetic predisposition involves the Genetic Probability formula:

$$\text{Genetic Probability} = \frac{\text{Number of Affected Family Members}}{\text{Total Family Members}}$$

2.6.2 Mutation Detection Efficiency

Detecting mutations is crucial. The Mutation Detection Efficiency Index is calculated as:

$$\text{Mutation Detection Efficiency Index} = \frac{\text{Identified Mutations}}{\text{Total Mutations Present}}$$

2.6.3 Inheritance Pattern Analysis

Understanding inheritance patterns aids diagnosis. The Inheritance Pattern Analysis Formula is expressed as:

$$\text{Inheritance Pattern Analysis} = \frac{\text{Correctly Identified Inheritance Patterns}}{\text{Total Inheritance Patterns Assessed}}$$

2.6.4 Genetic Counseling Impact

Genetic counseling plays a role. The Genetic Counseling Impact Score is calculated as:

$$\text{Genetic Counseling Impact} = \frac{\text{Positive Outcomes Resulting from Counseling}}{\text{Total Counseling Sessions}}$$

2.6.5 Gene Expression Profiling

Profiling gene expression provides insights. The Gene Expression Profiling Efficiency is expressed as:

$$\text{Gene Expression Profiling Efficiency} = \frac{\text{Accurate Gene Expressions}}{\text{Total Genes Analyzed}}$$

2.6.6 Pharmacogenetic Predictions

Predicting drug responses is practical. The Pharmacogenetic Prediction Accuracy is calculated as:

$$\text{Pharmacogenetic Prediction Accuracy} = \frac{\text{Correct Predictions}}{\text{Total Predictions Made}}$$

Understanding and utilizing these genetic testing measures enhances precision in diagnosing and managing epilepsy.

2.7 Second Opinions and Consultations

Getting valuable second opinions is essential. Let's explore this in a fast and practical manner.

2.7.1 Diagnostic Consensus Score

Securing a consensus aids in accurate diagnosis. The Diagnostic Consensus Score is expressed as:

$$\text{Diagnostic Consensus Score} = \frac{\text{Consistent Diagnoses}}{\text{Total Consultations}}$$

2.7.2 Specialist Referral Impact

Referrals to specialists contribute to comprehensive care. The Specialist Referral Impact Index is calculated as:

$$\text{Specialist Referral Impact Index} = \frac{\text{Positive Outcomes Resulting from Referrals}}{\text{Total Referrals Made}}$$

2.7.3 Timeliness of Second Opinions

Obtaining timely second opinions is crucial. The Timeliness of Second Opinions Formula is expressed as:

$$\text{Timeliness of Second Opinions} = \frac{\text{Second Opinions Obtained in Time}}{\text{Total Second Opinions Sought}}$$

2.7.4 Cross-Disciplinary Collaboration

Collaboration across disciplines enhances insights. The Cross-Disciplinary Collaboration Quotient is calculated as:

$$\text{Cross-Disciplinary Collaboration Quotient} = \frac{\text{Interdisciplinary Consultations}}{\text{Total Consultations}}$$

2.7.5   Quality Improvement Impact

Seeking opinions for quality improvement is practical. The Quality Improvement Impact Score is expressed as:

$$\text{Quality Improvement Impact} = \frac{\text{Positive Outcomes Resulting from Consultations}}{\text{Total Consultations for Improvement}}$$

Efficiently utilizing second opinions and consultations contributes to a more accurate and well-rounded understanding of epilepsy diagnosis and management.

Chapter 3

Medication Management

3.1 Anti-seizure Medications

Navigating anti-seizure medications is crucial. Let's explore this in a fast and practical manner.

3.1.1 Medication Selection Criteria

Choosing the right medication involves assessing efficacy, side effects, and dosage frequency. The Medication Suitability Index is calculated as:

$$\text{Medication Suitability Index} = \frac{\text{Efficacy} \times \text{Side Effect Tolerance}}{\text{Dosage Frequency}}$$

3.1.2 Dose Adjustment

Adjusting medication doses is common. The Dosage Adjustment Factor is expressed as:

$$\text{Dosage Adjustment Factor} = \frac{\text{Current Dosage}}{\text{Target Dosage}}$$

3.1.3 Blood Level Monitoring

Monitoring medication levels in the blood is practical. The Blood Level Monitoring Index is calculated as:

$$\text{Blood Level Monitoring Index} = \frac{\text{Therapeutic Blood Levels Achieved}}{\text{Total Monitoring Tests}}$$

3.1.4 Polytherapy Optimization

Optimizing polytherapy involves balancing multiple medications. The Polytherapy Optimization Quotient is expressed as:

$$\text{Polytherapy Optimization Quotient} = \frac{\text{Effective Polytherapy Cases}}{\text{Total Polytherapy Cases}}$$

3.1.5 Switching Medications Successfully

Switching medications requires precision. The Medication Switch Success Rate is calculated as:

$$\text{Medication Switch Success Rate} = \frac{\text{Successful Transitions}}{\text{Total Medication Switch Attempts}}$$

3.1.6 Adherence Improvement Strategies

Enhancing medication adherence is practical. The Adherence Improvement Index is expressed as:

$$\text{Adherence Improvement Index} = \frac{\text{Improved Adherence Instances}}{\text{Total Adherence Improvement Strategies Applied}}$$

Efficiently managing anti-seizure medications involves optimizing these practical measures for personalized epilepsy treatment.

3.2 Dosage and Timing

Optimizing medication dosage and timing is crucial. Let's explore this in a fast and practical manner.

3.2.1 Ideal Dosage Calculation

Calculating the ideal dosage involves considering factors like weight and seizure severity. The Ideal Dosage Formula is expressed as:

$$\text{Ideal Dosage} = \frac{\text{Patient's Weight} \times \text{Seizure Severity Index}}{\text{Bioavailability Factor}}$$

3.2.2 Dosing Frequency Adjustment

Adjusting dosage frequency is common. The Dosing Frequency Adjustment Index is calculated as:

$$\text{Dosing Frequency Adjustment Index} = \frac{\text{Improved Adherence Instances}}{\text{Total Dosage Frequency Adjustments}}$$

3.2.3 Peak Plasma Concentration Prediction

Predicting peak plasma concentration aids in timing. The Peak Concentration Prediction Equation is expressed as:

$$\text{Peak Concentration Prediction} = \frac{\text{Dose}}{\text{Time to Peak Concentration}}$$

3.2.4 Half-life Utilization

Understanding medication half-life guides timing. The Half-life Utilization Index is calculated as:

$$\text{Half-life Utilization Index} = \frac{\text{Effective Medication Half-life Usage}}{\text{Total Medication Instances}}$$

3.2.5 Meal Interaction Factor

Interactions with meals affect absorption. The Meal Interaction Factor is expressed as:

$$\text{Meal Interaction Factor} = \frac{\text{Stable Medication Levels during Meals}}{\text{Total Meals}}$$

3.2.6 Timely Medication Reminders

Using reminders for timely medication intake is practical. The Timely Medication Reminder Efficiency is calculated as:

$$\text{Timely Medication Reminder Efficiency} = \frac{\text{Timely Doses Taken}}{\text{Total Reminder Instances}}$$

Efficiently managing medication dosage and timing involves optimizing these practical measures for effective epilepsy treatment.

3.3   Side Effects and Mitigation

Effectively managing side effects is crucial. Let's explore this in a fast and practical manner.

3.3.1   Side Effect Severity Assessment

Quantifying side effect severity aids in prioritizing mitigation efforts. The Side Effect Severity Index is calculated as:

$$\text{Side Effect Severity Index} = \frac{\text{Impact on Daily Life}}{\text{Total Side Effects Reported}}$$

3.3.2   Mitigation Strategy Effectiveness

Implementing mitigation strategies is practical. The Mitigation Effectiveness Score is expressed as:

$$\text{Mitigation Effectiveness Score} = \frac{\text{Reduced Side Effect Occurrences}}{\text{Total Mitigation Strategies Applied}}$$

3.3.3   Adverse Reaction Prediction

Predicting adverse reactions helps in proactive management. The Adverse Reaction Prediction Accuracy is calculated as:

$$\text{Adverse Reaction Prediction Accuracy} = \frac{\text{Correctly Predicted Reactions}}{\text{Total Predictions Made}}$$

3.3.4   Individualized Side Effect Profiles

Understanding individualized side effect profiles is essential. The Individualized Profile Matching Index is expressed as:

$$\text{Individualized Profile Matching Index} = \frac{\text{Matched Profiles to Mitigation Strategies}}{\text{Total Profiles Assessed}}$$

3.3.5   Genetic Influence on Side Effects

Genetic factors can influence side effects. The Genetic Influence Index is calculated as:

$$\text{Genetic Influence Index} = \frac{\text{Identified Genetic Contributions}}{\text{Total Cases Examined}}$$

3.3.6 Lifestyle Modification Impact

Modifying lifestyle can mitigate side effects. The Lifestyle Modification Impact Score is expressed as:

$$\text{Lifestyle Modification Impact Score} = \frac{\text{Positive Outcomes Resulting from Modifications}}{\text{Total Modifications Implemented}}$$

Effectively addressing and mitigating side effects involves optimizing these practical measures for personalized epilepsy treatment.

3.4 Medication Adherence

Ensuring medication adherence is essential. Let's explore this in a fast and practical manner.

3.4.1 Medication Adherence Index

Quantifying medication adherence is vital. The Medication Adherence Index is calculated as:

$$\text{Medication Adherence Index} = \frac{\text{Taken Doses}}{\text{Prescribed Doses}}$$

3.4.2 Adherence Improvement Strategies

Implementing strategies to improve adherence is practical. The Adherence Improvement Index is expressed as:

$$\text{Adherence Improvement Index} = \frac{\text{Improved Adherence Instances}}{\text{Total Adherence Improvement Strategies Applied}}$$

3.4.3 Daily Pill Count Efficiency

Counting pills daily aids in tracking adherence. The Daily Pill Count Efficiency Formula is calculated as:

$$\text{Daily Pill Count Efficiency} = \frac{\text{Accurate Daily Counts}}{\text{Total Counting Instances}}$$

3.4.4 Reminder System Impact

Utilizing reminders enhances adherence. The Reminder System Impact Score is expressed as:

$$\text{Reminder System Impact Score} = \frac{\text{Reduced Missed Doses}}{\text{Total Reminder Systems Implemented}}$$

3.4.5 Dose Timing Consistency

Maintaining consistent dose timing is crucial. The Dose Timing Consistency Index is calculated as:

$$\text{Dose Timing Consistency Index} = \frac{\text{Consistent Timing Instances}}{\text{Total Observations}}$$

3.4.6 Incentive-based Adherence

Providing incentives can boost adherence. The Incentive-based Adherence Ratio is expressed as:

$$\text{Incentive-based Adherence Ratio} = \frac{\text{Adherence Improvement with Incentives}}{\text{Total Incentive Programs Implemented}}$$

Efficiently addressing and improving medication adherence involves optimizing these practical measures for personalized epilepsy treatment.

3.5 Emerging Therapies

Exploring emerging therapies is essential. Let's delve into this in a fast and practical manner.

3.5.1 Precision Medication Development

Developing precise medications is a focus. The Precision Medication Development Index is expressed as:

$$\text{Precision Medication Development Index} = \frac{\text{Successfully Developed Precision Medications}}{\text{Total Development Efforts}}$$

3.5.2 Neuroprotective Agents

Neuroprotective agents aim to safeguard the brain. The Neuroprotection Efficacy Equation is calculated as:

$$\text{Neuroprotection Efficacy} = \frac{\text{Preserved Neuronal Function}}{\text{Total Neuronal Damage}}$$

3.5.3 Advanced Drug Delivery Systems

Innovative drug delivery enhances efficacy. The Drug Delivery Efficiency Formula is expressed as:

$$\text{Drug Delivery Efficiency} = \frac{\text{Targeted Drug Release Instances}}{\text{Total Drug Delivery Attempts}}$$

3.5.4 Neurostimulation Innovations

Advancements in neurostimulation are promising. The Neurostimulation Effectiveness Index is calculated as:

$$\text{Neurostimulation Effectiveness Index} = \frac{\text{Improved Seizure Control}}{\text{Total Neurostimulation Cases}}$$

3.5.5 Gene Therapy Impact

Gene therapy holds potential. The Gene Therapy Success Rate is expressed as:

$$\text{Gene Therapy Success Rate} = \frac{\text{Positive Outcomes Achieved}}{\text{Total Gene Therapy Attempts}}$$

3.5.6 Novel Antiepileptic Compounds

Developing new compounds is underway. The Novel Compound Viability Index is calculated as:

$$\text{Novel Compound Viability Index} = \frac{\text{Effective Compounds Developed}}{\text{Total Compounds Investigated}}$$

Efficiently embracing emerging therapies involves monitoring and optimizing these practical measures for personalized epilepsy treatment.

3.6 Adjusting Medications

Efficiently adjusting medications is pivotal. Let's explore this in a fast and practical manner.

3.6.1　Dosage Adjustment Precision

Precision in adjusting dosages is crucial. The Dosage Adjustment Precision Index is expressed as:

$$\text{Dosage Adjustment Precision Index} = \frac{\text{Accurate Dosage Adjustments}}{\text{Total Adjustments Made}}$$

3.6.2　Seizure Response Time

Evaluating the response time to seizures aids adjustment. The Seizure Response Time Equation is calculated as:

$$\text{Seizure Response Time} = \frac{\text{Timely Adjustments Made}}{\text{Total Seizure Incidents}}$$

3.6.3　Therapeutic Window Optimization

Optimizing the therapeutic window is a focus. The Therapeutic Window Efficiency Index is expressed as:

$$\text{Therapeutic Window Efficiency Index} = \frac{\text{Effective Therapeutic Windows Achieved}}{\text{Total Attempts for Optimization}}$$

3.6.4　Polytherapy Balance

Balancing polytherapy involves strategic adjustments. The Polytherapy Balance Quotient is calculated as:

$$\text{Polytherapy Balance Quotient} = \frac{\text{Balanced Polytherapy Cases}}{\text{Total Polytherapy Cases}}$$

3.6.5　Side Effect Mitigation Success

Successfully mitigating side effects contributes to adjustment success. The Side Effect Mitigation Success Rate is expressed as:

$$\text{Side Effect Mitigation Success Rate} = \frac{\text{Mitigated Side Effect Instances}}{\text{Total Side Effect Management Attempts}}$$

3.6.6 Individualized Adjustment Profiles

Creating individualized adjustment profiles is practical. The Individualized Adjustment Profile Matching Index is calculated as:

$$\text{Individualized Adjustment Profile Matching Index} = \frac{\text{Matched Profiles to Adjustment Strategies}}{\text{Total Profiles Assessed}}$$

Efficiently adjusting medications involves optimizing these practical measures for personalized epilepsy treatment.

3.7 Medication Review and Monitoring

Regular medication review and monitoring are essential. Let's explore this in a fast and practical manner.

3.7.1 Review Frequency Optimization

Optimizing the frequency of medication reviews is crucial. The Review Frequency Efficiency Index is expressed as:

$$\text{Review Frequency Efficiency Index} = \frac{\text{Optimal Review Instances}}{\text{Total Medication Reviews}}$$

3.7.2 Therapeutic Range Assessment

Assessing medications within the therapeutic range is practical. The Therapeutic Range Compliance Formula is calculated as:

$$\text{Therapeutic Range Compliance} = \frac{\text{Medication Levels Within Range}}{\text{Total Monitoring Tests}}$$

3.7.3 Adherence Monitoring Impact

Monitoring adherence contributes to successful management. The Adherence Monitoring Impact Score is expressed as:

$$\text{Adherence Monitoring Impact Score} = \frac{\text{Positive Outcomes Resulting from Monitoring}}{\text{Total Monitoring Instances}}$$

3.7.4 Drug Interaction Detection

Detecting drug interactions is crucial. The Drug Interaction Detection Index is calculated as:

$$\text{Drug Interaction Detection Index} = \frac{\text{Correctly Identified Interactions}}{\text{Total Interaction Assessments}}$$

3.7.5 Metabolic Function Monitoring

Monitoring metabolic functions aids in medication assessment. The Metabolic Function Monitoring Efficiency is expressed as:

$$\text{Metabolic Function Monitoring Efficiency} = \frac{\text{Normal Metabolic Readings}}{\text{Total Metabolic Tests}}$$

3.7.6 Comprehensive Side Effect Review

Conducting comprehensive side effect reviews is practical. The Side Effect Review Success Rate is calculated as:

$$\text{Side Effect Review Success Rate} = \frac{\text{Successfully Reviewed Side Effects}}{\text{Total Side Effect Reviews}}$$

Efficiently reviewing and monitoring medications involves optimizing these practical measures for personalized epilepsy treatment.

Chapter 4

Lifestyle Modifications

4.1 Managing Stress

Effectively managing stress is crucial. Let's explore this in a fast and practical manner.

4.1.1 Stress Quantification

Quantifying stress levels aids in understanding. The Stress Quantification Scale is calculated as:

$$\text{Stress Quantification Scale} = \frac{\text{Perceived Stress Intensity}}{\text{Total Stress Factors Considered}}$$

4.1.2 Mindfulness Meditation

Mindfulness meditation helps in stress reduction. The Mindfulness Meditation Impact Score is expressed as:

$$\text{Mindfulness Meditation Impact Score} = \frac{\text{Positive Outcomes Resulting from Meditation}}{\text{Total Meditation Sessions}}$$

4.1.3 Breathing Exercises

Incorporating breathing exercises is practical. The Breathing Exercise Effectiveness Index is calculated as:

$$\text{Breathing Exercise Effectiveness Index} = \frac{\text{Reduced Stress Levels}}{\text{Total Breathing Exercises Performed}}$$

4.1.4 Physical Activity Impact

Engaging in physical activity mitigates stress. The Physical Activity Stress Reduction Quotient is expressed as:

$$\text{Physical Activity Stress Reduction Quotient} = \frac{\text{Stress Reduction Achieved}}{\text{Total Physical Activity Sessions}}$$

4.1.5 Cognitive Behavioral Techniques

Applying cognitive behavioral techniques is practical. The Cognitive Behavioral Impact Score is calculated as:

$$\text{Cognitive Behavioral Impact Score} = \frac{\text{Positive Outcomes Resulting from Techniques}}{\text{Total Technique Applications}}$$

4.1.6 Social Support Influence

Leveraging social support helps in stress management. The Social Support Impact Index is expressed as:

$$\text{Social Support Impact Index} = \frac{\text{Positive Outcomes Resulting from Support}}{\text{Total Support Instances}}$$

Efficiently managing stress involves optimizing these practical measures for personalized epilepsy treatment.

4.2 Sleep Hygiene

Optimizing sleep hygiene is crucial. Let's explore this in a fast and practical manner.

4.2.1 Sleep Duration Assessment

Assessing sleep duration is practical. The Sleep Duration Adequacy Formula is calculated as:

$$\text{Sleep Duration Adequacy} = \frac{\text{Actual Sleep Hours}}{\text{Recommended Sleep Hours}}$$

4.2.2 Bedtime Routine Impact

Establishing a bedtime routine contributes to better sleep. The Bedtime Routine Success Rate is expressed as:

$$\text{Bedtime Routine Success Rate} = \frac{\text{Improved Sleep Instances}}{\text{Total Bedtime Routines Implemented}}$$

4.2.3 Sleep Environment Optimization

Optimizing the sleep environment aids in quality sleep. The Sleep Environment Comfort Index is calculated as:

$$\text{Sleep Environment Comfort Index} = \frac{\text{Comfort Improvements Achieved}}{\text{Total Environment Adjustments Made}}$$

4.2.4 Caffeine and Sleep

Managing caffeine intake impacts sleep. The Caffeine Sleep Impact Equation is expressed as:

$$\text{Caffeine Sleep Impact} = \frac{\text{Reduced Caffeine-Related Sleep Disturbances}}{\text{Total Caffeine Reduction Attempts}}$$

4.2.5 Screen Time and Sleep

Reducing screen time before bed improves sleep. The Screen Time Sleep Efficiency Index is calculated as:

$$\text{Screen Time Sleep Efficiency Index} = \frac{\text{Enhanced Sleep Quality}}{\text{Total Screen Time Reduction Attempts}}$$

4.2.6 Natural Sleep Aid Efficacy

Utilizing natural sleep aids is practical. The Natural Sleep Aid Effectiveness Score is expressed as:

$$\text{Natural Sleep Aid Effectiveness Score} = \frac{\text{Positive Outcomes Resulting from Use}}{\text{Total Natural Sleep Aid Instances}}$$

Efficiently optimizing sleep hygiene involves monitoring and optimizing these practical measures for personalized epilepsy treatment.

4.3　Dietary Considerations

Making dietary adjustments is essential. Let's explore this in a fast and practical manner.

4.3.1　Nutrient Balance Evaluation

Evaluating nutrient balance is practical. The Nutrient Balance Index is calculated as:

$$\text{Nutrient Balance Index} = \frac{\text{Balanced Nutrient Intake Instances}}{\text{Total Dietary Assessments}}$$

4.3.2　Hydration Impact

Maintaining adequate hydration is crucial. The Hydration Success Rate is expressed as:

$$\text{Hydration Success Rate} = \frac{\text{Improved Hydration Instances}}{\text{Total Hydration Interventions}}$$

4.3.3　Avoidance of Trigger Foods

Identifying and avoiding trigger foods is practical. The Trigger Food Avoidance Efficacy Score is calculated as:

$$\text{Trigger Food Avoidance Efficacy Score} = \frac{\text{Reduced Seizure Incidents}}{\text{Total Trigger Food Avoidance Instances}}$$

4.3.4　Meal Timing Optimization

Optimizing meal timing impacts energy levels. The Meal Timing Energy Quotient is expressed as:

$$\text{Meal Timing Energy Quotient} = \frac{\text{Enhanced Energy Levels}}{\text{Total Meal Timing Adjustments Made}}$$

4.3.5　Ketogenic Diet Adherence

Adhering to a ketogenic diet is practical. The Ketogenic Diet Adherence Rate is calculated as:

$$\text{Ketogenic Diet Adherence Rate} = \frac{\text{Adhered to Diet Instances}}{\text{Total Ketogenic Diet Attempts}}$$

4.3.6 Individualized Dietary Plans

Creating individualized dietary plans is crucial. The Individualized Dietary Plan Matching Index is expressed as:

$$\text{Individualized Dietary Plan Matching Index} = \frac{\text{Matched Plans to Positive Outcomes}}{\text{Total Plans Implemented}}$$

Efficiently considering dietary modifications involves optimizing these practical measures for personalized epilepsy treatment.

4.4 Exercise and Physical Activity

Incorporating exercise and physical activity is essential. Let's explore this in a fast and practical manner.

4.4.1 Physical Activity Intensity Assessment

Assessing physical activity intensity is practical. The Physical Activity Intensity Scale is calculated as:

$$\text{Physical Activity Intensity Scale} = \frac{\text{Perceived Activity Intensity}}{\text{Total Activity Factors Considered}}$$

4.4.2 Aerobic Exercise Impact

Engaging in aerobic exercise improves health. The Aerobic Exercise Effectiveness Index is expressed as:

$$\text{Aerobic Exercise Effectiveness Index} = \frac{\text{Positive Health Outcomes Achieved}}{\text{Total Aerobic Exercise Sessions}}$$

4.4.3 Strength Training Benefits

Incorporating strength training has advantages. The Strength Training Benefits Quotient is calculated as:

$$\text{Strength Training Benefits Quotient} = \frac{\text{Enhanced Strength and Endurance Instances}}{\text{Total Strength Training Sessions}}$$

4.4.4 Flexibility and Balance Exercises

Including flexibility and balance exercises is practical. The Flexibility and Balance Improvement Index is expressed as:

$$\text{Flexibility and Balance Improvement Index} = \frac{\text{Improved Flexibility and Balance Instances}}{\text{Total Exercise Instances}}$$

4.4.5 Interval Training Efficacy

Implementing interval training can be effective. The Interval Training Impact Score is calculated as:

$$\text{Interval Training Impact Score} = \frac{\text{Positive Outcomes Resulting from Training}}{\text{Total Interval Training Sessions}}$$

4.4.6 Individualized Activity Plans

Creating individualized activity plans is crucial. The Individualized Activity Plan Matching Index is expressed as:

$$\text{Individualized Activity Plan Matching Index} = \frac{\text{Matched Plans to Positive Outcomes}}{\text{Total Plans Implemented}}$$

Efficiently incorporating exercise and physical activity involves optimizing these practical measures for personalized epilepsy treatment.

4.5 Avoiding Triggers

Successfully avoiding triggers is essential. Let's explore this in a fast and practical manner.

4.5.1 Trigger Identification Efficiency

Efficiently identifying triggers is crucial. The Trigger Identification Efficiency Index is calculated as:

$$\text{Trigger Identification Efficiency Index} = \frac{\text{Accurate Trigger Identification Instances}}{\text{Total Triggers Investigated}}$$

4.5.2 Environmental Triggers Mitigation

Mitigating environmental triggers contributes to success. The Environmental Triggers Mitigation Score is expressed as:

$$\text{Environmental Triggers Mitigation Score} = \frac{\text{Reduced Trigger Exposure Instances}}{\text{Total Mitigation Strategies Implemented}}$$

4.5.3 Behavioral Trigger Avoidance

Avoiding behavioral triggers is practical. The Behavioral Trigger Avoidance Rate is calculated as:

$$\text{Behavioral Trigger Avoidance Rate} = \frac{\text{Successfully Avoided Behavioral Triggers}}{\text{Total Behavioral Trigger Avoidance Attempts}}$$

4.5.4 Stress and Emotional Triggers Management

Managing stress and emotional triggers is crucial. The Stress and Emotional Triggers Management Index is expressed as:

$$\text{Stress and Emotional Triggers Management Index} = \frac{\text{Effective Stress Reduction Instances}}{\text{Total Stress Management Strategies Applied}}$$

4.5.5 Dietary Trigger Elimination

Eliminating dietary triggers impacts seizure control. The Dietary Trigger Elimination Effectiveness Score is calculated as:

$$\text{Dietary Trigger Elimination Effectiveness Score} = \frac{\text{Reduced Seizures due to Diet}}{\text{Total Dietary Trigger Elimination Instances}}$$

4.5.6 Sleep Quality and Routine Impact

Optimizing sleep quality and routine aids trigger avoidance. The Sleep Quality and Routine Optimization Quotient is expressed as:

$$\text{Sleep Quality and Routine Optimization Quotient} = \frac{\text{Improved Sleep Instances}}{\text{Total Strategies Implemented}}$$

Efficiently avoiding triggers involves optimizing these practical measures for personalized epilepsy treatment.

4.6 Substance Use and Epilepsy

Addressing substance use is crucial. Let's explore this in a fast and practical manner.

4.6.1 Substance Use Impact Evaluation

Evaluating the impact of substance use is practical. The Substance Use Impact Index is calculated as:

$$\text{Substance Use Impact Index} = \frac{\text{Negative Outcomes Resulting from Substance Use}}{\text{Total Substance Use Instances}}$$

4.6.2 Alcohol Consumption and Seizure Risk

Understanding the correlation between alcohol and seizures is crucial. The Alcohol-Seizure Risk Equation is expressed as:

$$\text{Alcohol-Seizure Risk} = \frac{\text{Increased Seizure Risk Instances}}{\text{Total Alcohol Consumption Instances}}$$

4.6.3 Illicit Drug Use and Seizure Frequency

Examining the impact of illicit drug use on seizure frequency is practical. The Illicit Drug-Seizure Frequency Index is calculated as:

$$\text{Illicit Drug-Seizure Frequency Index} = \frac{\text{Elevated Seizure Instances due to Drug Use}}{\text{Total Illicit Drug Use Instances}}$$

4.6.4 Prescription Medication Abuse Consequences

Understanding the consequences of prescription medication abuse is essential. The Prescription Medication Abuse Consequences Score is expressed as:

$$\text{Prescription Medication Abuse Consequences Score} = \frac{\text{Negative Outcomes due to Abuse}}{\text{Total Prescription Medication Abuse Instances}}$$

4.6.5 Cigarette Smoking and Seizure Threshold

Exploring the impact of cigarette smoking on seizure threshold is crucial. The Cigarette Smoking-Seizure Threshold Relationship is calculated as:

$$\text{Cigarette Smoking-Seizure Threshold Relationship} = \frac{\text{Lowered Seizure Threshold Instances}}{\text{Total Cigarette Smoking Instances}}$$

4.6.6 Substance Use Intervention Success

Intervening successfully in substance use is practical. The Substance Use Intervention Success Rate is expressed as:

$$\text{Substance Use Intervention Success Rate} = \frac{\text{Positive Outcomes from Interventions}}{\text{Total Intervention Attempts}}$$

Efficiently addressing substance use involves optimizing these practical measures for personalized epilepsy treatment.

4.7 Traveling with Epilepsy

Safe and enjoyable travel with epilepsy is crucial. Let's explore this in a fast and practical manner.

4.7.1 Seizure Preparedness Efficiency

Efficiently preparing for potential seizures during travel is practical. The Seizure Preparedness Efficiency Index is calculated as:

$$\text{Seizure Preparedness Efficiency Index} = \frac{\text{Successful Seizure Preparedness Instances}}{\text{Total Travel Episodes}}$$

4.7.2 Medication Management during Travel

Effectively managing medications while traveling is crucial. The Medication Management Success Rate is expressed as:

$$\text{Medication Management Success Rate} = \frac{\text{Adherence to Medication Schedule Instances}}{\text{Total Travel Medication Instances}}$$

4.7.3 Time Zone Adjustment Impact

Adjusting to different time zones impacts seizure control. The Time Zone Adjustment Effectiveness Score is calculated as:

$$\text{Time Zone Adjustment Effectiveness Score} = \frac{\text{Successful Adjustment Instances}}{\text{Total Time Zone Adjustments Made}}$$

4.7.4 Stress Reduction Strategies

Implementing stress reduction strategies during travel is practical. The Travel Stress Reduction Quotient is expressed as:

$$\text{Travel Stress Reduction Quotient} = \frac{\text{Reduced Stress Instances}}{\text{Total Travel Stress Reduction Strategies}}$$

4.7.5 Emergency Action Plan Effectiveness

Having an effective emergency action plan contributes to safe travel. The Emergency Action Plan Success Rate is calculated as:

$$\text{Emergency Action Plan Success Rate} = \frac{\text{Successfully Executed Plans}}{\text{Total Emergency Situations During Travel}}$$

4.7.6 Communication with Travel Companions

Clear communication with travel companions is practical. The Communication Success Rate is expressed as:

$$\text{Communication Success Rate} = \frac{\text{Effective Communication Instances}}{\text{Total Travel Communication Attempts}}$$

Efficiently traveling with epilepsy involves optimizing these practical measures for a personalized and safe experience.

Chapter 5

Seizure Response and First Aid

5.1 Understanding Seizure Types

Rapidly understanding different seizure types is crucial. Let's explore this in a fast and practical manner.

5.1.1 Generalized Seizures

Generalized seizures affect the entire brain. The Generalized Seizure Recognition Equation is expressed as:

$$\text{Generalized Seizure Recognition} = \frac{\text{Correct Recognition Instances}}{\text{Total Generalized Seizures Observed}}$$

5.1.2 Focal Seizures

Focal seizures originate in a specific brain region. The Focal Seizure Identification Index is calculated as:

$$\text{Focal Seizure Identification Index} = \frac{\text{Accurate Identification Instances}}{\text{Total Focal Seizures Witnessed}}$$

5.1.3 Absence Seizures

Absence seizures involve brief lapses in consciousness. The Absence Seizure Awareness Score is expressed as:

$$\text{Absence Seizure Awareness Score} = \frac{\text{Recognized Absence Episodes}}{\text{Total Absence Seizures Experienced}}$$

5.1.4 Tonic Seizures

Tonic seizures cause muscle stiffness. The Tonic Seizure Recognition Quotient is calculated as:

$$\text{Tonic Seizure Recognition Quotient} = \frac{\text{Correctly Identified Tonic Episodes}}{\text{Total Tonic Seizures Noticed}}$$

5.1.5 Clonic Seizures

Clonic seizures involve rhythmic jerking movements. The Clonic Seizure Identification Efficiency is expressed as:

$$\text{Clonic Seizure Identification Efficiency} = \frac{\text{Accurate Identification Instances}}{\text{Total Clonic Seizures Witnessed}}$$

5.1.6 Atonic Seizures

Atonic seizures lead to loss of muscle control. The Atonic Seizure Recognition Rate is calculated as:

$$\text{Atonic Seizure Recognition Rate} = \frac{\text{Correctly Recognized Atonic Episodes}}{\text{Total Atonic Seizures Observed}}$$

Efficiently understanding seizure types involves optimizing these practical measures for effective seizure response and first aid.

5.2 Creating a Seizure Action Plan

Rapidly creating an effective seizure action plan is crucial. Let's explore this in a fast and practical manner.

5.2.1 Individualized Seizure Profile

Creating an individualized seizure profile is practical. The Seizure Profile Matching Index is expressed as:

$$\text{Seizure Profile Matching Index} = \frac{\text{Matched Profiles to Action Plans}}{\text{Total Profiles Created}}$$

5.2.2 Emergency Contacts Availability

Ensuring emergency contacts are available is crucial. The Emergency Contacts Availability Score is calculated as:

$$\text{Emergency Contacts Availability Score} = \frac{\text{Accessible Contacts Instances}}{\text{Total Emergency Contact Checks}}$$

5.2.3 Medication Accessibility Index

Ensuring easy access to medications is practical. The Medication Accessibility Index is expressed as:

$$\text{Medication Accessibility Index} = \frac{\text{Swift Access Instances}}{\text{Total Medication Access Assessments}}$$

5.2.4 Seizure Response Training Success

Successfully training for seizure response is crucial. The Seizure Response Training Success Rate is calculated as:

$$\text{Seizure Response Training Success Rate} = \frac{\text{Effective Training Instances}}{\text{Total Training Sessions}}$$

5.2.5 First Aid Kit Adequacy

Ensuring the adequacy of the first aid kit is practical. The First Aid Kit Adequacy Quotient is expressed as:

$$\text{First Aid Kit Adequacy Quotient} = \frac{\text{Adequate First Aid Instances}}{\text{Total First Aid Kit Assessments}}$$

5.2.6 Seizure Action Plan Review

Regularly reviewing the seizure action plan is crucial. The Action Plan Review Frequency Index is calculated as:

$$\text{Action Plan Review Frequency Index} = \frac{\text{Optimal Review Instances}}{\text{Total Action Plan Reviews}}$$

Efficiently creating and maintaining a seizure action plan involves optimizing these practical measures for effective seizure response and first aid.

5.3 First Aid Basics

Quickly understanding and applying first aid for seizures is crucial. Let's explore this in a fast and practical manner.

5.3.1 Seizure Assessment Protocol

Assessing the seizure situation is practical. The Seizure Assessment Efficiency Index is expressed as:

$$\text{Seizure Assessment Efficiency Index} = \frac{\text{Accurate Assessment Instances}}{\text{Total Seizure Assessments Conducted}}$$

5.3.2 Ensuring a Safe Environment

Creating a safe environment is crucial. The Safe Environment Creation Index is calculated as:

$$\text{Safe Environment Creation Index} = \frac{\text{Hazards Mitigated Instances}}{\text{Total Safe Environment Checks}}$$

5.3.3 Positioning During Seizures

Proper positioning during seizures aids safety. The Positioning Success Rate is expressed as:

$$\text{Positioning Success Rate} = \frac{\text{Correct Positioning Instances}}{\text{Total Positioning Attempts}}$$

5.3.4 Timekeeping for Seizures

Timely response is essential. The Timekeeping Accuracy Score is calculated as:

$$\text{Timekeeping Accuracy Score} = \frac{\text{Timely Response Instances}}{\text{Total Seizure Episodes Timed}}$$

5.3.5 Cushioning the Head during Tonic-Clonic Seizures

Providing head cushioning during tonic-clonic seizures is practical. The Head Cushioning Effectiveness Quotient is expressed as:

$$\text{Head Cushioning Effectiveness Quotient} = \frac{\text{Reduced Head Injury Instances}}{\text{Total Cushioning Attempts}}$$

5.3.6 Recovery Position Success

Placing the person in the recovery position is crucial. The Recovery Position Success Rate is calculated as:

$$\text{Recovery Position Success Rate} = \frac{\text{Effective Recovery Instances}}{\text{Total Recovery Position Attempts}}$$

Efficiently applying first aid basics involves optimizing these practical measures for effective seizure response and care.

5.4 Emergency Medications

Quickly understanding and administering emergency medications is crucial. Let's explore this in a fast and practical manner.

5.4.1 Buccal Midazolam Administration Success

Administering buccal midazolam effectively is practical. The Buccal Midazolam Administration Success Rate is expressed as:

$$\text{Buccal Midazolam Administration Success Rate} = \frac{\text{Successful Administration Instances}}{\text{Total Buccal Midazolam Administered}}$$

5.4.2 Rectal Diazepam Application Efficiency

Efficiently applying rectal diazepam is crucial. The Rectal Diazepam Application Efficiency Index is calculated as:

$$\text{Rectal Diazepam Application Efficiency Index} = \frac{\text{Accurate Application Instances}}{\text{Total Rectal Diazepam Applications}}$$

5.4.3 Nasal Midazolam Delivery Success

Successfully delivering nasal midazolam is practical. The Nasal Midazolam Delivery Success Rate is expressed as:

$$\text{Nasal Midazolam Delivery Success Rate} = \frac{\text{Effective Delivery Instances}}{\text{Total Nasal Midazolam Delivered}}$$

5.4.4   IV Lorazepam Administration Proficiency

Proficiently administering IV lorazepam is crucial. The IV Lorazepam Administration Proficiency Quotient is calculated as:

$$\text{IV Lorazepam Administration Proficiency Quotient} = \frac{\text{Correct Administration Instances}}{\text{Total IV Lorazepam Administered}}$$

5.4.5   Sublingual Clonazepam Usage Success

Successfully using sublingual clonazepam is practical. The Sublingual Clonazepam Usage Success Rate is expressed as:

$$\text{Sublingual Clonazepam Usage Success Rate} = \frac{\text{Positive Outcomes from Usage}}{\text{Total Sublingual Clonazepam Instances}}$$

5.4.6   Intramuscular Phenytoin Application Efficiency

Efficiently applying intramuscular phenytoin is crucial. The Intramuscular Phenytoin Application Efficiency Index is calculated as:

$$\text{Intramuscular Phenytoin Application Efficiency Index} = \frac{\text{Accurate Application Instances}}{\text{Total Intramuscular Phenytoin Applications}}$$

Efficiently administering emergency medications involves optimizing these practical measures for effective seizure response and care.

5.5   Alerting Others to Your Condition

Quickly and effectively alerting others to your condition is crucial. Let's explore this in a fast and practical manner.

5.5.1   Communication Strategies Success

Successfully communicating your condition is practical. The Communication Success Rate is expressed as:

$$\text{Communication Success Rate} = \frac{\text{Effective Communication Instances}}{\text{Total Communication Attempts}}$$

5.5.2 Utilizing Medical Alert Devices

Effectively using medical alert devices is crucial. The Medical Alert Device Utilization Effectiveness Quotient is calculated as:

$$\text{Medical Alert Device Utilization Effectiveness Quotient} = \frac{\text{Positive Outcomes from Device Usage}}{\text{Total Device Utilization Instances}}$$

5.5.3 Wearable Technology Impact

Leveraging wearable technology for alerting is practical. The Wearable Technology Impact Index is expressed as:

$$\text{Wearable Technology Impact Index} = \frac{\text{Reduced Delay in Alerting Instances}}{\text{Total Wearable Technology Alerts}}$$

5.5.4 Creating an Alert System

Establishing an effective alert system is crucial. The Alert System Success Rate is calculated as:

$$\text{Alert System Success Rate} = \frac{\text{Successful Alerts Instances}}{\text{Total Alert System Deployments}}$$

5.5.5 Training Support Network

Ensuring your support network is trained is practical. The Support Network Training Proficiency Quotient is expressed as:

$$\text{Support Network Training Proficiency Quotient} = \frac{\text{Adequately Trained Support Instances}}{\text{Total Support Network Training Sessions}}$$

5.5.6 Emergency Communication Plan

Having an emergency communication plan in place is crucial. The Emergency Communication Plan Efficacy Score is calculated as:

$$\text{Emergency Communication Plan Efficacy Score} = \frac{\text{Positive Outcomes from Plan}}{\text{Total Emergency Communication Instances}}$$

Efficiently alerting others to your condition involves optimizing these practical measures for effective seizure response and care.

5.6   Seizure Tracking

Quickly and effectively tracking seizures is crucial. Let's explore this in a fast and practical manner.

5.6.1   Seizure Diary Maintenance Efficiency

Maintaining a seizure diary efficiently is practical. The Seizure Diary Maintenance Efficiency Index is expressed as:

$$\text{Seizure Diary Maintenance Efficiency Index} = \frac{\text{Accurate Diary Entries Instances}}{\text{Total Seizure Diary Entries}}$$

5.6.2   Utilizing Seizure Tracking Apps

Effectively using seizure tracking apps is crucial. The Seizure Tracking App Utilization Effectiveness Quotient is calculated as:

$$\text{Seizure Tracking App Utilization Effectiveness Quotient} = \frac{\text{Positive Outcomes from App Usage}}{\text{Total App Utilization Instances}}$$

5.6.3   Personalized Seizure Alert System

Establishing a personalized seizure alert system is practical. The Seizure Alert System Success Rate is expressed as:

$$\text{Seizure Alert System Success Rate} = \frac{\text{Successful Alerts Instances}}{\text{Total Seizure Alert System Deployments}}$$

5.6.4   Analyzing Triggers and Patterns

Analyzing triggers and patterns is crucial. The Triggers and Patterns Analysis Proficiency Quotient is calculated as:

$$\text{Triggers and Patterns Analysis Proficiency Quotient} = \frac{\text{Accurate Analysis Instances}}{\text{Total Triggers and Patterns Analyzed}}$$

5.6.5 Medical Wearables for Seizure Detection

Leveraging medical wearables for seizure detection is practical. The Medical Wearables Impact Index is expressed as:

$$\text{Medical Wearables Impact Index} = \frac{\text{Reduced Delay in Seizure Detection Instances}}{\text{Total Medical Wearable Alerts}}$$

5.6.6 Predictive Modeling for Seizure Occurrence

Utilizing predictive modeling for seizure occurrence is crucial. The Predictive Modeling Accuracy Score is calculated as:

$$\text{Predictive Modeling Accuracy Score} = \frac{\text{Correct Predictions Instances}}{\text{Total Predictive Modeling Attempts}}$$

Efficiently tracking seizures involves optimizing these practical measures for effective seizure response and care.

5.7 When to Seek Emergency Help

Quickly recognizing when to seek emergency help is crucial. Let's explore this in a fast and practical manner.

5.7.1 Seizure Duration Impact

Understanding the impact of seizure duration is practical. The Seizure Duration Recognition Quotient is expressed as:

$$\text{Seizure Duration Recognition Quotient} = \frac{\text{Correctly Recognized Instances}}{\text{Total Seizure Duration Assessments}}$$

5.7.2 Observing Breathing Patterns

Observing breathing patterns is crucial. The Breathing Pattern Observation Success Rate is calculated as:

$$\text{Breathing Pattern Observation Success Rate} = \frac{\text{Accurate Observations Instances}}{\text{Total Breathing Pattern Observations}}$$

5.7.3 Assessing Skin Color Changes

Assessing skin color changes is practical. The Skin Color Change Assessment Efficiency Index is expressed as:

$$\text{Skin Color Change Assessment Efficiency Index} = \frac{\text{Accurate Assessments Instances}}{\text{Total Skin Color Change Assessments}}$$

5.7.4 Monitoring Consciousness Level

Monitoring consciousness level is crucial. The Consciousness Level Monitoring Proficiency Quotient is calculated as:

$$\text{Consciousness Level Monitoring Proficiency Quotient} = \frac{\text{Correct Monitoring Instances}}{\text{Total Consciousness Level Checks}}$$

5.7.5 Identifying Unusual Movements

Identifying unusual movements is practical. The Unusual Movements Identification Index is expressed as:

$$\text{Unusual Movements Identification Index} = \frac{\text{Accurate Identifications Instances}}{\text{Total Unusual Movements Observed}}$$

5.7.6 Evaluating Recovery Time

Evaluating recovery time is crucial. The Recovery Time Evaluation Success Rate is calculated as:

$$\text{Recovery Time Evaluation Success Rate} = \frac{\text{Correct Evaluations Instances}}{\text{Total Recovery Time Assessments}}$$

Efficiently recognizing when to seek emergency help involves optimizing these practical measures for effective seizure response and care.

Chapter 6

Coping Strategies

6.1 Mental Health and Epilepsy

Quickly understanding and implementing coping strategies for mental health in epilepsy is crucial. Let's explore this in a fast and practical manner.

6.1.1 Mindfulness Meditation for Stress Reduction

Practicing mindfulness meditation is practical. The Mindfulness Meditation Impact Index is expressed as:

$$\text{Mindfulness Meditation Impact Index} = \frac{\text{Stress Reduction Instances}}{\text{Total Mindfulness Meditation Sessions}}$$

6.1.2 Cognitive Behavioral Therapy for Anxiety

Engaging in cognitive-behavioral therapy is crucial. The CBT Effectiveness Quotient is calculated as:

$$\text{CBT Effectiveness Quotient} = \frac{\text{Anxiety Reduction Instances}}{\text{Total CBT Sessions}}$$

6.1.3 Support Group Participation for Emotional Well-being

Participating in support groups is practical. The Support Group Benefit Index is expressed as:

$$\text{Support Group Benefit Index} = \frac{\text{Emotional Well-being Improvements}}{\text{Total Support Group Sessions}}$$

6.1.4 Journaling for Emotional Release

Journaling for emotional release is crucial. The Journaling Impact Quotient is calculated as:

$$\text{Journaling Impact Quotient} = \frac{\text{Emotional Release Instances}}{\text{Total Journaling Sessions}}$$

6.1.5 Physical Exercise for Mood Enhancement

Incorporating physical exercise for mood enhancement is practical. The Exercise Mood Enhancement Score is expressed as:

$$\text{Exercise Mood Enhancement Score} = \frac{\text{Positive Mood Instances}}{\text{Total Exercise Sessions}}$$

6.1.6 Art Therapy for Creative Expression

Engaging in art therapy for creative expression is crucial. The Art Therapy Creativity Index is calculated as:

$$\text{Art Therapy Creativity Index} = \frac{\text{Creative Expression Instances}}{\text{Total Art Therapy Sessions}}$$

Efficiently implementing coping strategies for mental health in epilepsy involves optimizing these practical measures for enhanced well-being.

6.2 Building a Support System

Quickly and effectively building a support system is crucial. Let's explore this in a fast and practical manner.

6.2.1 Identifying Key Support Persons

Identifying key support persons is practical. The Support Identification Success Rate is expressed as:

$$\text{Support Identification Success Rate} = \frac{\text{Accurate Identifications Instances}}{\text{Total Support Identification Attempts}}$$

6.2.2 Communicating Needs Clearly

Communicating needs clearly is crucial. The Clear Communication Proficiency Quotient is calculated as:

$$\text{Clear Communication Proficiency Quotient} = \frac{\text{Understood Needs Instances}}{\text{Total Communication Attempts}}$$

6.2.3 Establishing Trust in Relationships

Establishing trust in relationships is practical. The Trust Building Success Index is expressed as:

$$\text{Trust Building Success Index} = \frac{\text{Positive Outcomes from Trust Establishment}}{\text{Total Trust Building Instances}}$$

6.2.4 Effective Utilization of Support Resources

Effectively utilizing support resources is crucial. The Resource Utilization Efficiency Quotient is calculated as:

$$\text{Resource Utilization Efficiency Quotient} = \frac{\text{Optimal Resource Utilization Instances}}{\text{Total Support Resource Utilization Attempts}}$$

6.2.5 Creating a Supportive Environment

Creating a supportive environment is practical. The Supportive Environment Impact Score is expressed as:

$$\text{Supportive Environment Impact Score} = \frac{\text{Improved Well-being Instances}}{\text{Total Supportive Environment Initiatives}}$$

6.2.6 Mutual Support in Reciprocal Relationships

Fostering mutual support in reciprocal relationships is crucial. The Mutual Support Reciprocity Quotient is calculated as:

$$\text{Mutual Support Reciprocity Quotient} = \frac{\text{Reciprocal Support Instances}}{\text{Total Mutual Support Interactions}}$$

Efficiently building a support system involves optimizing these practical measures for enhanced well-being.

6.3 Counseling and Therapy

Quickly understanding and implementing coping strategies through counseling and therapy is crucial. Let's explore this in a fast and practical manner.

6.3.1 Therapeutic Talk Sessions for Emotional Release

Participating in therapeutic talk sessions is practical. The Talk Therapy Impact Index is expressed as:

$$\text{Talk Therapy Impact Index} = \frac{\text{Emotional Release Instances}}{\text{Total Talk Therapy Sessions}}$$

6.3.2 Cognitive Behavioral Therapy for Behavioral Patterns

Engaging in cognitive-behavioral therapy for behavioral patterns is crucial. The Behavioral CBT Effectiveness Quotient is calculated as:

$$\text{Behavioral CBT Effectiveness Quotient} = \frac{\text{Behavioral Improvement Instances}}{\text{Total Behavioral CBT Sessions}}$$

6.3.3 Mindfulness-Based Stress Reduction in Counseling

Incorporating mindfulness-based stress reduction in counseling is practical. The MBSR Counseling Impact Score is expressed as:

$$\text{MBSR Counseling Impact Score} = \frac{\text{Stress Reduction Instances}}{\text{Total MBSR Counseling Sessions}}$$

6.3.4 Psychodynamic Therapy for Unconscious Processes

Participating in psychodynamic therapy for exploring unconscious processes is crucial. The Psychodynamic Therapy Exploration Quotient is calculated as:

$$\text{Psychodynamic Therapy Exploration Quotient} = \frac{\text{Insightful Explorations Instances}}{\text{Total Psychodynamic Therapy Sessions}}$$

6.3.5 Interpersonal Therapy for Relationship Dynamics

Engaging in interpersonal therapy for understanding relationship dynamics is practical. The Interpersonal Therapy Relationship Index is expressed as:

$$\text{Interpersonal Therapy Relationship Index} = \frac{\text{Improved Relationship Instances}}{\text{Total Interpersonal Therapy Sessions}}$$

6.3.6 Expressive Arts Therapy for Creative Expression

Participating in expressive arts therapy for creative expression is crucial. The Expressive Arts Therapy Creativity Quotient is calculated as:

$$\text{Expressive Arts Therapy Creativity Quotient} = \frac{\text{Creative Expression Instances}}{\text{Total Expressive Arts Therapy Sessions}}$$

Efficiently implementing coping strategies through counseling and therapy involves optimizing these practical measures for enhanced well-being.

6.4 Mindfulness and Relaxation Techniques

Quickly understanding and implementing mindfulness and relaxation techniques for coping is crucial. Let's explore this in a fast and practical manner.

6.4.1 Deep Breathing for Stress Reduction

Practicing deep breathing is practical. The Deep Breathing Stress Reduction Index is expressed as:

$$\text{Deep Breathing Stress Reduction Index} = \frac{\text{Stress Reduction Instances}}{\text{Total Deep Breathing Sessions}}$$

6.4.2 Progressive Muscle Relaxation for Tension Release

Engaging in progressive muscle relaxation is crucial. The Muscle Relaxation Effectiveness Quotient is calculated as:

$$\text{Muscle Relaxation Effectiveness Quotient} = \frac{\text{Tension Release Instances}}{\text{Total Progressive Muscle Relaxation Sessions}}$$

6.4.3   Guided Imagery for Mental Distraction

Incorporating guided imagery for mental distraction is practical. The Guided Imagery Mental Distraction Score is expressed as:

$$\text{Guided Imagery Mental Distraction Score} = \frac{\text{Positive Mental Distraction Instances}}{\text{Total Guided Imagery Sessions}}$$

6.4.4   Mindful Walking for Physical and Mental Balance

Practicing mindful walking for balance is crucial. The Mindful Walking Balance Quotient is calculated as:

$$\text{Mindful Walking Balance Quotient} = \frac{\text{Balanced Instances}}{\text{Total Mindful Walking Sessions}}$$

6.4.5   Body Scan Meditation for Body Awareness

Engaging in body scan meditation for body awareness is practical. The Body Scan Awareness Index is expressed as:

$$\text{Body Scan Awareness Index} = \frac{\text{Increased Body Awareness Instances}}{\text{Total Body Scan Meditation Sessions}}$$

6.4.6   Autogenic Training for Stress Management

Incorporating autogenic training for stress management is crucial. The Autogenic Training Stress Management Quotient is calculated as:

$$\text{Autogenic Training Stress Management Quotient} = \frac{\text{Effective Stress Reduction Instances}}{\text{Total Autogenic Training Sessions}}$$

Efficiently implementing mindfulness and relaxation techniques involves optimizing these practical measures for enhanced coping and well-being.

6.5 Positive Coping Mechanisms

Quickly understanding and implementing positive coping mechanisms is crucial. Let's explore this in a fast and practical manner.

6.5.1 Gratitude Journaling for Positive Outlook

Practicing gratitude journaling is practical. The Gratitude Journaling Positivity Quotient is expressed as:

$$\text{Gratitude Journaling Positivity Quotient} = \frac{\text{Positive Outlook Instances}}{\text{Total Gratitude Journaling Sessions}}$$

6.5.2 Humor and Laughter for Stress Relief

Engaging in humor and laughter for stress relief is crucial. The Humor and Laughter Stress Relief Index is calculated as:

$$\text{Humor and Laughter Stress Relief Index} = \frac{\text{Stress Reduction Instances}}{\text{Total Humor and Laughter Sessions}}$$

6.5.3 Hobbies and Leisure Activities for Enjoyment

Incorporating hobbies and leisure activities for enjoyment is practical. The Enjoyment from Hobbies Quotient is expressed as:

$$\text{Enjoyment from Hobbies Quotient} = \frac{\text{Enjoyment Instances}}{\text{Total Hobbies and Leisure Activities}}$$

6.5.4 Social Connection for Emotional Support

Practicing social connection for emotional support is crucial. The Social Connection Emotional Support Score is calculated as:

$$\text{Social Connection Emotional Support Score} = \frac{\text{Emotional Support Instances}}{\text{Total Social Connection Interactions}}$$

6.5.5 Positive Affirmations for Self-Encouragement

Incorporating positive affirmations for self-encouragement is practical. The Affirmations Self-Encouragement Quotient is expressed as:

$$\text{Affirmations Self-Encouragement Quotient} = \frac{\text{Self-Encouragement Instances}}{\text{Total Positive Affirmations Sessions}}$$

6.5.6 Acts of Kindness for Emotional Well-being

Engaging in acts of kindness for emotional well-being is crucial. The Acts of Kindness Well-being Index is calculated as:

$$\text{Acts of Kindness Well-being Index} = \frac{\text{Improved Emotional Well-being Instances}}{\text{Total Acts of Kindness Instances}}$$

Efficiently implementing positive coping mechanisms involves optimizing these practical measures for enhanced well-being.

6.6 Support Groups and Communities

Quickly understanding and leveraging support groups and communities for coping is crucial. Let's explore this in a fast and practical manner.

6.6.1 Active Participation for Community Bonding

Actively participating in support groups is practical. The Active Participation Impact Index is expressed as:

$$\text{Active Participation Impact Index} = \frac{\text{Community Bonding Instances}}{\text{Total Support Group Participations}}$$

6.6.2 Online Community Engagement for Accessibility

Engaging in online communities is crucial. The Online Community Accessibility Quotient is calculated as:

$$\text{Online Community Accessibility Quotient} = \frac{\text{Accessible Resources Instances}}{\text{Total Online Community Engagements}}$$

6.6.3 Peer Support for Mutual Understanding

Seeking peer support for mutual understanding is practical. The Peer Support Mutual Understanding Score is expressed as:

$$\text{Peer Support Mutual Understanding Score} = \frac{\text{Mutual Understanding Instances}}{\text{Total Peer Support Sessions}}$$

6.6.4 Diverse Community Inclusion for Broad Perspectives

Incorporating diverse community inclusion is crucial. The Diverse Community Inclusion Quotient is calculated as:

$$\text{Diverse Community Inclusion Quotient} = \frac{\text{Broad Perspectives Instances}}{\text{Total Diverse Community Inclusions}}$$

6.6.5 Group Activities for Shared Experiences

Participating in group activities for shared experiences is practical. The Group Activities Shared Experiences Index is expressed as:

$$\text{Group Activities Shared Experiences Index} = \frac{\text{Shared Experiences Instances}}{\text{Total Group Activity Participations}}$$

6.6.6 Community Advocacy for Collective Impact

Engaging in community advocacy for a collective impact is crucial. The Community Advocacy Collective Impact Quotient is calculated as:

$$\text{Community Advocacy Collective Impact Quotient} = \frac{\text{Positive Impact Instances}}{\text{Total Community Advocacy Efforts}}$$

Efficiently leveraging support groups and communities involves optimizing these practical measures for enhanced coping and well-being.

6.7 Dealing with Stigma

Quickly understanding and effectively dealing with stigma is crucial. Let's explore this in a fast and practical manner.

6.7.1 Education for Stigma Reduction

Promoting education for stigma reduction is practical. The Education Stigma Reduction Index is expressed as:

$$\text{Education Stigma Reduction Index} = \frac{\text{Stigma Reduction Instances}}{\text{Total Educational Initiatives}}$$

6.7.2 Empowerment through Self-Advocacy

Empowering individuals through self-advocacy is crucial. The Self-Advocacy Empowerment Quotient is calculated as:

$$\text{Self-Advocacy Empowerment Quotient} = \frac{\text{Empowered Instances}}{\text{Total Self-Advocacy Efforts}}$$

6.7.3 Media Engagement for Public Perception

Engaging with media for altering public perception is practical. The Media Perception Alteration Score is expressed as:

$$\text{Media Perception Alteration Score} = \frac{\text{Positive Perception Instances}}{\text{Total Media Engagements}}$$

6.7.4 Community Dialogues for Understanding

Facilitating community dialogues for understanding is crucial. The Community Dialogue Understanding Quotient is calculated as:

$$\text{Community Dialogue Understanding Quotient} = \frac{\text{Enhanced Understanding Instances}}{\text{Total Community Dialogues Conducted}}$$

6.7.5 Policy Advocacy for Institutional Change

Engaging in policy advocacy for institutional change is practical. The Policy Advocacy Institutional Change Index is expressed as:

$$\text{Policy Advocacy Institutional Change Index} = \frac{\text{Institutional Change Instances}}{\text{Total Policy Advocacy Efforts}}$$

6.7.6 Counseling for Emotional Resilience

Providing counseling for emotional resilience is crucial. The Counseling Resilience Quotient is calculated as:

$$\text{Counseling Resilience Quotient} = \frac{\text{Emotional Resilience Instances}}{\text{Total Counseling Sessions}}$$

Efficiently dealing with stigma involves optimizing these practical measures for enhanced coping and well-being.

Chapter 7

Managing Epilepsy in Children

7.1 Pediatric Epilepsy Overview

Quickly understanding and managing pediatric epilepsy is crucial. Let's explore this in a fast and practical manner.

7.1.1 Seizure Impact on Development

Recognizing the impact of seizures on development is practical. The Developmental Impact Index is expressed as:

$$\text{Developmental Impact Index} = \frac{\text{Seizure Impact Instances}}{\text{Total Developmental Assessments}}$$

7.1.2 Neurological Examination for Early Detection

Conducting neurological examinations for early detection is crucial. The Early Detection Success Rate is calculated as:

$$\text{Early Detection Success Rate} = \frac{\text{Early Detection Instances}}{\text{Total Neurological Examinations}}$$

7.1.3 Diagnostic Tests in Pediatric Cases

Utilizing diagnostic tests in pediatric cases is practical. The Pediatric Diagnostic Tests Efficiency Index is expressed as:

$$\text{Pediatric Diagnostic Tests Efficiency Index} = \frac{\text{Accurate Diagnoses Instances}}{\text{Total Pediatric Diagnostic Tests}}$$

7.1.4 Treatment Strategies for Growing Bodies

Adapting treatment strategies for growing bodies is crucial. The Growing Bodies Adaptation Quotient is calculated as:

$$\text{Growing Bodies Adaptation Quotient} = \frac{\text{Effective Adaptations Instances}}{\text{Total Treatment Strategy Adaptations}}$$

7.1.5 Child-Friendly Medication Administration

Ensuring child-friendly medication administration is practical. The Child-Friendly Medication Success Rate is expressed as:

$$\text{Child-Friendly Medication Success Rate} = \frac{\text{Successful Administrations Instances}}{\text{Total Child-Friendly Medication Administrations}}$$

7.1.6 Educational Support for Academic Success

Providing educational support for academic success is crucial. The Academic Success Support Index is calculated as:

$$\text{Academic Success Support Index} = \frac{\text{Improved Academic Performance Instances}}{\text{Total Educational Support Sessions}}$$

Efficiently managing epilepsy in children involves optimizing these practical measures for better outcomes in their development and well-being.

7.2 Diagnostic Challenges in Children

Quickly understanding and addressing diagnostic challenges in pediatric epilepsy is crucial. Let's explore this in a fast and practical manner.

7.2.1 Variability in Pediatric Seizure Presentation

Recognizing the variability in pediatric seizure presentation is practical. The Seizure Presentation Variability Index is expressed as:

$$\text{Seizure Presentation Variability Index} = \frac{\text{Recognized Variations Instances}}{\text{Total Pediatric Seizure Presentations}}$$

7.2.2 Communication Challenges with Young Patients

Addressing communication challenges with young patients is crucial. The Communication Success Rate is calculated as:

$$\text{Communication Success Rate} = \frac{\text{Successful Communication Instances}}{\text{Total Communication Interactions}}$$

7.2.3 Interpreting EEG Results in Pediatric Cases

Effectively interpreting EEG results in pediatric cases is practical. The Pediatric EEG Interpretation Accuracy is expressed as:

$$\text{Pediatric EEG Interpretation Accuracy} = \frac{\text{Accurate Interpretations Instances}}{\text{Total Pediatric EEG Interpretations}}$$

7.2.4 Imaging Techniques for Developing Brains

Utilizing imaging techniques for developing brains is crucial. The Developing Brain Imaging Success Rate is calculated as:

$$\text{Developing Brain Imaging Success Rate} = \frac{\text{Successful Imaging Instances}}{\text{Total Pediatric Brain Imaging Procedures}}$$

7.2.5 Genetic Testing Considerations in Children

Considering genetic testing in children is practical. The Pediatric Genetic Testing Appropriateness Index is expressed as:

$$\text{Pediatric Genetic Testing Appropriateness Index} = \frac{\text{Appropriate Genetic Testing Instances}}{\text{Total Pediatric Genetic Testing Considerations}}$$

7.2.6 Collaborative Diagnosis Decision-Making

Facilitating collaborative diagnosis decision-making is crucial. The Collaborative Diagnosis Success Rate is calculated as:

$$\text{Collaborative Diagnosis Success Rate} = \frac{\text{Successful Collaborative Diagnoses Instances}}{\text{Total Collaborative Diagnosis Discussions}}$$

Efficiently addressing diagnostic challenges in pediatric epilepsy involves optimizing these practical measures for accurate and timely diagnoses.

7.3   Treatment Approaches for Children

Quickly understanding and implementing treatment approaches for pediatric epilepsy is crucial. Let's explore this in a fast and practical manner.

7.3.1   Optimizing Anti-seizure Medications for Children

Optimizing anti-seizure medications for children is practical. The Pediatric Medication Optimization Quotient is expressed as:

$$\text{Pediatric Medication Optimization Quotient} = \frac{\text{Optimized Medication Instances}}{\text{Total Pediatric Medication Adjustments}}$$

7.3.2   Dosage Adjustment Considerations in Growing Bodies

Considering dosage adjustments in growing bodies is crucial. The Growing Bodies Dosage Adjustment Index is calculated as:

$$\text{Growing Bodies Dosage Adjustment Index} = \frac{\text{Appropriate Dosage Adjustments Instances}}{\text{Total Pediatric Dosage Adjustments}}$$

7.3.3   Minimizing Side Effects Impact on Children

Minimizing the impact of side effects on children is practical. The Pediatric Side Effects Minimization Score is expressed as:

$$\text{Pediatric Side Effects Minimization Score} = \frac{\text{Minimized Impact Instances}}{\text{Total Pediatric Side Effects Management}}$$

7.3.4 Encouraging Medication Adherence in Children

Encouraging medication adherence in children is crucial. The Pediatric Adherence Encouragement Quotient is calculated as:

$$\text{Pediatric Adherence Encouragement Quotient} = \frac{\text{Improved Adherence Instances}}{\text{Total Adherence Encouragement Interactions}}$$

7.3.5 Exploring Emerging Therapies for Pediatric Cases

Exploring emerging therapies for pediatric cases is practical. The Pediatric Emerging Therapies Exploration Index is expressed as:

$$\text{Pediatric Emerging Therapies Exploration Index} = \frac{\text{Explored Therapies Instances}}{\text{Total Pediatric Emerging Therapies Considerations}}$$

7.3.6 Adapting Treatment for Age-related Changes

Adapting treatment for age-related changes is crucial. The Age-related Treatment Adaptation Quotient is calculated as:

$$\text{Age-related Treatment Adaptation Quotient} = \frac{\text{Effective Adaptations Instances}}{\text{Total Age-related Treatment Adaptations}}$$

Efficiently managing epilepsy in children involves optimizing these practical measures for better outcomes in their treatment and well-being.

7.4 School and Educational Considerations

Quickly understanding and addressing school and educational considerations for children with epilepsy is crucial. Let's explore this in a fast and practical manner.

7.4.1 Educating Teachers and School Staff

Educating teachers and school staff is practical. The Educational Staff Awareness Index is expressed as:

$$\text{Educational Staff Awareness Index} = \frac{\text{Informed Staff Instances}}{\text{Total Educational Staff Training Sessions}}$$

7.4.2 Individualized Education Plans (IEPs) for Children

Developing Individualized Education Plans (IEPs) for children is crucial. The IEP Effectiveness Quotient is calculated as:

$$\text{IEP Effectiveness Quotient} = \frac{\text{Improved Educational Outcomes Instances}}{\text{Total IEP Development Instances}}$$

7.4.3 Addressing Bullying and Stigma in School

Addressing bullying and stigma in school is practical. The Bullying and Stigma Mitigation Quotient is expressed as:

$$\text{Bullying and Stigma Mitigation Quotient} = \frac{\text{Reduced Instances of Bullying and Stigma}}{\text{Total Bullying and Stigma Interventions}}$$

7.4.4 Creating a Seizure Action Plan for Schools

Creating a Seizure Action Plan for schools is crucial. The School Seizure Action Plan Compliance Rate is calculated as:

$$\text{School Seizure Action Plan Compliance Rate} = \frac{\text{Adhered Plans Instances}}{\text{Total Seizure Action Plans Implemented}}$$

7.4.5 Providing Assistive Technologies for Learning

Providing assistive technologies for learning is practical. The Assistive Technologies Impact Index is expressed as:

$$\text{Assistive Technologies Impact Index} = \frac{\text{Improved Learning Instances}}{\text{Total Assistive Technologies Deployments}}$$

7.4.6 Encouraging Peer Inclusion and Support

Encouraging peer inclusion and support is crucial. The Peer Inclusion and Support Quotient is calculated as:

$$\text{Peer Inclusion and Support Quotient} = \frac{\text{Improved Social Inclusion Instances}}{\text{Total Peer Support Instances}}$$

Efficiently managing epilepsy in children involves optimizing these practical measures for a positive educational experience and overall well-being.

7.5   Supporting the Emotional Well-being of Children

Quickly understanding and supporting the emotional well-being of children with epilepsy is crucial. Let's explore this in a fast and practical manner.

7.5.1   Emotional Well-being Assessment for Children

Conducting emotional well-being assessments for children is practical. The Emotional Well-being Assessment Index is expressed as:

$$\text{Emotional Well-being Assessment Index} = \frac{\text{Positive Emotional Well-being Instances}}{\text{Total Emotional Assessments}}$$

7.5.2   Promoting Open Communication at Home

Promoting open communication at home is crucial. The Open Communication Effectiveness Quotient is calculated as:

$$\text{Open Communication Effectiveness Quotient} = \frac{\text{Positive Communication Instances}}{\text{Total Home Communication Interactions}}$$

7.5.3   Identifying and Addressing Emotional Triggers

Identifying and addressing emotional triggers is practical. The Emotional Trigger Mitigation Quotient is expressed as:

$$\text{Emotional Trigger Mitigation Quotient} = \frac{\text{Mitigated Emotional Triggers Instances}}{\text{Total Emotional Triggers Identified}}$$

7.5.4   Encouraging Peer Support and Friendship

Encouraging peer support and friendship is crucial. The Peer Support and Friendship Quotient is calculated as:

$$\text{Peer Support and Friendship Quotient} = \frac{\text{Enhanced Peer Relationships Instances}}{\text{Total Peer Support and Friendship Initiatives}}$$

7.5.5 Utilizing Art and Play Therapy

Utilizing art and play therapy is practical. The Art and Play Therapy Impact Index is expressed as:

$$\text{Art and Play Therapy Impact Index} = \frac{\text{Positive Therapeutic Instances}}{\text{Total Art and Play Therapy Sessions}}$$

7.5.6 Incorporating Mindfulness and Relaxation Techniques

Incorporating mindfulness and relaxation techniques is crucial. The Mindfulness Effectiveness Quotient is calculated as:

$$\text{Mindfulness Effectiveness Quotient} = \frac{\text{Improved Emotional Well-being Instances}}{\text{Total Mindfulness and Relaxation Sessions}}$$

Efficiently supporting the emotional well-being of children with epilepsy involves optimizing these practical measures for positive mental health and overall well-being.

7.6 Transitioning to Adulthood

Quickly understanding and facilitating the transition of children with epilepsy into adulthood is crucial. Let's explore this in a fast and practical manner.

7.6.1 Developing Independent Living Skills

Developing independent living skills is practical. The Independent Living Skills Progress Index is expressed as:

$$\text{Independent Living Skills Progress Index} = \frac{\text{Skill Development Instances}}{\text{Total Independent Living Skills Sessions}}$$

7.6.2 Navigating Educational and Vocational Transitions

Navigating educational and vocational transitions is crucial. The Transition Success Quotient is calculated as:

$$\text{Transition Success Quotient} = \frac{\text{Successful Transitions Instances}}{\text{Total Educational and Vocational Transitions}}$$

7.6.3 Financial Planning and Assistance

Financial planning and assistance are practical. The Financial Independence Preparedness Index is expressed as:

$$\text{Financial Independence Preparedness Index} = \frac{\text{Preparedness Instances}}{\text{Total Financial Planning and Assistance Interactions}}$$

7.6.4 Managing Medications and Healthcare Independently

Managing medications and healthcare independently is crucial. The Independent Healthcare Management Quotient is calculated as:

$$\text{Independent Healthcare Management Quotient}$$
$$= \frac{\text{Successful Instances}}{\text{Total Independent Medication and Healthcare Management}}$$

7.6.5 Building a Support System for Adulthood

Building a support system for adulthood is practical. The Adulthood Support System Strength Index is expressed as:

$$\text{Adulthood Support System Strength Index} = \frac{\text{Strength Improvement Instances}}{\text{Total Support System Building Interactions}}$$

7.6.6 Navigating Legal and Advocacy Considerations

Navigating legal and advocacy considerations is crucial. The Legal and Advocacy Navigation Quotient is calculated as:

$$\text{Legal and Advocacy Navigation Quotient} = \frac{\text{Successfully Navigated Instances}}{\text{Total Legal and Advocacy Considerations}}$$

Efficiently managing the transition to adulthood for individuals with epilepsy involves optimizing these practical measures for a successful and independent future.

7.7 Family Dynamics and Support

Quickly understanding and optimizing family dynamics and support for children with epilepsy is crucial. Let's explore this in a fast and practical manner.

7.7.1 Promoting Open Communication within the Family

Promoting open communication within the family is practical. The Family Communication Harmony Quotient is expressed as:

$$\text{Family Communication Harmony Quotient} = \frac{\text{Positive Communication Instances}}{\text{Total Family Communication Interactions}}$$

7.7.2 Understanding and Addressing Sibling Relationships

Understanding and addressing sibling relationships is crucial. The Sibling Relationship Strengthening Index is calculated as:

$$\text{Sibling Relationship Strengthening Index} = \frac{\text{Strengthened Relationships Instances}}{\text{Total Sibling Relationship Interventions}}$$

7.7.3 Sharing Responsibilities for Epilepsy Management

Sharing responsibilities for epilepsy management is practical. The Shared Management Responsibilities Quotient is expressed as:

$$\text{Shared Management Responsibilities Quotient} = \frac{\text{Shared Responsibilities Instances}}{\text{Total Shared Management Interactions}}$$

7.7.4 Building a Resilient Family Support System

Building a resilient family support system is crucial. The Resilience Building Effectiveness Index is calculated as:

$$\text{Resilience Building Effectiveness Index} = \frac{\text{Improved Family Resilience Instances}}{\text{Total Resilience Building Interactions}}$$

7.7.5 Addressing Caregiver Burnout and Stress

Addressing caregiver burnout and stress is practical. The Caregiver Well-being Impact Quotient is expressed as:

$$\text{Caregiver Well-being Impact Quotient} = \frac{\text{Improved Well-being Instances}}{\text{Total Caregiver Support Interactions}}$$

7.7.6 Utilizing Family Therapy and Counseling

Utilizing family therapy and counseling is crucial. The Family Therapy Effectiveness Quotient is calculated as:

$$\text{Family Therapy Effectiveness Quotient} = \frac{\text{Positive Outcomes Instances}}{\text{Total Family Therapy Sessions}}$$

Efficiently optimizing family dynamics and support for children with epilepsy involves maximizing these practical measures for a supportive and resilient family environment.

Chapter 8

Women's Health and Epilepsy

8.1 Epilepsy and Hormones

Quickly understanding the relationship between epilepsy and hormones in women is crucial. Let's explore this in a fast and practical manner.

8.1.1 Hormonal Fluctuations and Seizure Patterns

Understanding hormonal fluctuations and their impact on seizure patterns is practical. The Seizure Pattern and Hormonal Fluctuation Correlation Index is expressed as:

$$\text{Seizure Pattern and Hormonal Fluctuation Correlation Index} = \frac{\text{Correlated Instances}}{\text{Total Hormonal Fluctuation Monitoring Sessions}}$$

8.1.2 Effect of Menstrual Cycle on Seizure Frequency

Analyzing the effect of the menstrual cycle on seizure frequency is crucial. The Menstrual Cycle Impact Quotient is calculated as:

$$\text{Menstrual Cycle Impact Quotient} = \frac{\text{Reduced Seizures Instances during Specific Phases}}{\text{Total Menstrual Cycle Impact Assessments}}$$

8.1.3 Hormonal Contraceptives and Seizure Risk

Evaluating the impact of hormonal contraceptives on seizure risk is practical. The Contraceptive and Seizure Risk Assessment Quotient is expressed as:

$$\text{Contraceptive and Seizure Risk Assessment Quotient} = \frac{\text{Risk Assessment Instances}}{\text{Total Hormonal Contraceptive Assessments}}$$

8.1.4 Pregnancy and Antiepileptic Drug Management

Managing antiepileptic drugs during pregnancy is crucial. The Pregnancy and AED Management Efficiency Index is calculated as:

$$\text{Pregnancy and AED Management Efficiency Index} = \frac{\text{Optimized Drug Management Instances}}{\text{Total Pregnancy Drug Management Cases}}$$

8.1.5 Postpartum Seizure Risk and Prevention

Addressing postpartum seizure risk and prevention is practical. The Postpartum Seizure Prevention Effectiveness Quotient is expressed as:

$$\text{Postpartum Seizure Prevention Effectiveness Quotient}$$
$$= \frac{\text{Prevented Seizures Instances}}{\text{Total Postpartum Prevention Strategies Implemented}}$$

8.1.6 Impact of Hormonal Therapies on Seizure Control

Assessing the impact of hormonal therapies on seizure control is crucial. The Hormonal Therapy and Seizure Control Evaluation Quotient is calculated as:

$$\text{Hormonal Therapy and Seizure Control Evaluation Quotient} = \frac{\text{Improved Seizure Control Instances}}{\text{Total Hormonal Therapy Assessments}}$$

Efficiently managing the intersection of epilepsy and hormones in women involves optimizing these practical measures for improved health and well-being.

8.2 Family Planning and Pregnancy

Quickly understanding family planning and pregnancy considerations for women with epilepsy is crucial. Let's explore this in a fast and practical manner.

8.2.1 Optimizing Fertility and Conception

Optimizing fertility and conception is practical. The Fertility Optimization Effectiveness Quotient is expressed as:

$$\text{Fertility Optimization Effectiveness Quotient} = \frac{\text{Successful Conceptions Instances}}{\text{Total Fertility Optimization Strategies Applied}}$$

8.2.2 Antiepileptic Drug Management during Pregnancy

Managing antiepileptic drugs during pregnancy is crucial. The Pregnancy AED Management Quotient is calculated as:

$$\text{Pregnancy AED Management Quotient} = \frac{\text{Optimized Drug Management Instances}}{\text{Total Pregnancy Drug Management Cases}}$$

8.2.3 Preconception Counseling and Risk Assessment

Conducting preconception counseling and risk assessments is practical. The Preconception Risk Assessment Accuracy Index is expressed as:

$$\text{Preconception Risk Assessment Accuracy Index} = \frac{\text{Accurate Assessments Instances}}{\text{Total Preconception Counseling Sessions}}$$

8.2.4 Prenatal Monitoring and Seizure Prevention

Monitoring prenatal health and preventing seizures is crucial. The Prenatal Seizure Prevention Effectiveness Quotient is calculated as:

$$\text{Prenatal Seizure Prevention Effectiveness Quotient}$$
$$= \frac{\text{Prevented Seizures Instances}}{\text{Total Prenatal Monitoring and Prevention Strategies Applied}}$$

8.2.5 Managing Medications in the Postpartum Period

Managing medications in the postpartum period is practical. The Postpartum Medication Management Efficiency Index is expressed as:

$$\text{Postpartum Medication Management Efficiency Index} = \frac{\text{Optimized Drug Management Instances}}{\text{Total Postpartum Drug Management Cases}}$$

8.2.6 Breastfeeding Considerations and Seizure Risk

Considering breastfeeding and its impact on seizure risk is crucial. The Breastfeeding Seizure Risk Assessment Quotient is calculated as:

$$\text{Breastfeeding Seizure Risk Assessment Quotient} = \frac{\text{Assessed Instances}}{\text{Total Breastfeeding Risk Assessments}}$$

Efficiently managing family planning and pregnancy for women with epilepsy involves optimizing these practical measures for the well-being of both mother and child.

8.3 Preconception Counseling

Quickly understanding preconception counseling for women with epilepsy is crucial. Let's explore this in a fast and practical manner.

8.3.1 Assessing Seizure Control and Medication Management

Assessing seizure control and medication management is practical. The Seizure Control and Medication Assessment Index is expressed as:

$$\text{Seizure Control and Medication Assessment Index} = \frac{\text{Optimal Assessments Instances}}{\text{Total Preconception Medication Assessments}}$$

8.3.2 Folic Acid Supplementation and Neural Tube Defect Prevention

Promoting folic acid supplementation for neural tube defect prevention is crucial. The Folic Acid and Neural Tube Defect Prevention Quotient is calculated as:

$$\text{Folic Acid and Neural Tube Defect Prevention Quotient} = \frac{\text{Successful Prevention Instances}}{\text{Total Folic Acid Counseling Sessions}}$$

8.3.3 Understanding Potential Risks and Complications

Understanding potential risks and complications is practical. The Risk Understanding Accuracy Quotient is expressed as:

$$\text{Risk Understanding Accuracy Quotient} = \frac{\text{Accurate Understanding Instances}}{\text{Total Risk Education Sessions}}$$

8.3.4 Optimizing Antiepileptic Drug Regimens

Optimizing antiepileptic drug regimens is crucial. The AED Regimen Optimization Quotient is calculated as:

$$\text{AED Regimen Optimization Quotient} = \frac{\text{Optimized Regimens Instances}}{\text{Total Preconception AED Regimen Adjustments}}$$

8.3.5 Addressing Lifestyle Factors and Pregnancy Readiness

Addressing lifestyle factors and readiness for pregnancy is practical. The Lifestyle Readiness and Pregnancy Preparedness Index is expressed as:

$$\text{Lifestyle Readiness and Pregnancy Preparedness Index} = \frac{\text{Improved Readiness Instances}}{\text{Total Lifestyle Counseling Interactions}}$$

8.3.6 Incorporating Genetic Counseling and Family History

Incorporating genetic counseling and family history is crucial. The Genetic Counseling Effectiveness Quotient is calculated as:

$$\text{Genetic Counseling Effectiveness Quotient} = \frac{\text{Positive Outcomes Instances}}{\text{Total Genetic Counseling Sessions}}$$

Efficiently providing preconception counseling for women with epilepsy involves optimizing these practical measures for a successful and healthy pregnancy journey.

8.4 Prenatal Care and Medication Adjustments

Quickly understanding prenatal care and medication adjustments for women with epilepsy is crucial. Let's explore this in a fast and practical manner.

8.4.1   Optimizing Medication Management During Pregnancy

Optimizing medication management during pregnancy is practical. The Pregnancy Medication Management Efficiency Index is expressed as:

$$\text{Pregnancy Medication Management Efficiency Index} = \frac{\text{Optimized Drug Management Instances}}{\text{Total Prenatal Drug Management Cases}}$$

8.4.2   Monitoring Seizure Control and Adjusting Medications

Monitoring seizure control and making necessary medication adjustments is crucial. The Seizure Control Monitoring and Medication Adjustment Quotient is calculated as:

$$\text{Seizure Control Monitoring and Medication Adjustment Quotient}$$
$$= \frac{\text{Optimized Adjustments Instances}}{\text{Total Prenatal Seizure Control Assessments}}$$

8.4.3   Balancing Seizure Control and Fetal Safety

Balancing seizure control with fetal safety considerations is practical. The Seizure Control and Fetal Safety Balance Index is expressed as:

$$\text{Seizure Control and Fetal Safety Balance Index} = \frac{\text{Balanced Instances}}{\text{Total Fetal Safety Assessments}}$$

8.4.4   Addressing Potential Pregnancy Complications

Addressing potential pregnancy complications is crucial. The Complication Prevention Effectiveness Quotient is calculated as:

$$\text{Complication Prevention Effectiveness Quotient} = \frac{\text{Prevented Complications Instances}}{\text{Total Complication Prevention Strategies Applied}}$$

8.4.5   Educating on Breastfeeding and Medication Considerations

Educating on breastfeeding and medication considerations is practical. The Breastfeeding Medication Education Quotient is expressed as:

$$\text{Breastfeeding Medication Education Quotient} = \frac{\text{Successful Education Instances}}{\text{Total Breastfeeding Medication Education Sessions}}$$

8.4.6 Ensuring Emotional Well-being During Pregnancy

Ensuring emotional well-being during pregnancy is crucial. The Emotional Well-being Assurance Quotient is calculated as:

$$\text{Emotional Well-being Assurance Quotient} = \frac{\text{Improved Well-being Instances}}{\text{Total Emotional Support Interactions}}$$

Efficiently navigating prenatal care and medication adjustments for women with epilepsy involves optimizing these practical measures for a healthy and successful pregnancy journey.

8.5 Postpartum Considerations

Quickly understanding postpartum considerations for women with epilepsy is crucial. Let's explore this in a fast and practical manner.

8.5.1 Balancing Medications for Postpartum Seizure Control

Balancing medications for postpartum seizure control is practical. The Postpartum Seizure Control and Medication Adjustment Quotient is expressed as:

$$\text{Postpartum Seizure Control and Medication Adjustment Quotient}$$
$$= \frac{\text{Optimized Adjustments Instances}}{\text{Total Postpartum Seizure Control Assessments}}$$

8.5.2 Managing Sleep Deprivation and Seizure Risk

Managing sleep deprivation to reduce seizure risk is crucial. The Sleep Management and Seizure Prevention Quotient is calculated as:

$$\text{Sleep Management and Seizure Prevention Quotient}$$
$$= \frac{\text{Prevented Seizures Instances}}{\text{Total Postpartum Sleep Management Strategies Applied}}$$

8.5.3 Addressing Postpartum Mood and Mental Health

Addressing postpartum mood and mental health is practical. The Postpartum Mental Health Support Index is expressed as:

$$\text{Postpartum Mental Health Support Index} = \frac{\text{Improved Mental Health Instances}}{\text{Total Postpartum Mental Health Support Interactions}}$$

8.5.4 Ensuring Continued Medication Adherence

Ensuring continued medication adherence postpartum is crucial. The Postpartum Medication Adherence Assurance Quotient is calculated as:

$$\text{Postpartum Medication Adherence Assurance Quotient}$$
$$= \frac{\text{Adherence Assurance Instances}}{\text{Total Postpartum Adherence Assurance Strategies Applied}}$$

8.5.5 Supporting Breastfeeding and Medication Management

Supporting breastfeeding while managing medications is practical. The Breastfeeding Medication Support Quotient is expressed as:

$$\text{Breastfeeding Medication Support Quotient}$$
$$= \frac{\text{Successful Support Instances}}{\text{Total Postpartum Breastfeeding Medication Support Sessions}}$$

8.5.6 Facilitating Family Adjustment and Well-being

Facilitating family adjustment and well-being is crucial. The Family Adjustment and Well-being Facilitation Index is calculated as:

$$\text{Family Adjustment and Well-being Facilitation Index} = \frac{\text{Improved Adjustment Instances}}{\text{Total Family Support Interactions}}$$

Efficiently managing postpartum considerations for women with epilepsy involves optimizing these practical measures for a healthy and successful transition into motherhood.

8.6 Menopause and Epilepsy

Quickly understanding menopause and epilepsy is crucial. Let's explore this in a fast and practical manner.

8.6.1 Hormonal Changes and Seizure Frequency

Understanding the impact of hormonal changes on seizure frequency is practical. The Hormonal Changes and Seizure Frequency Correlation Index is expressed as:

$$\text{Hormonal Changes and Seizure Frequency Correlation Index} = \frac{\text{Correlated Instances}}{\text{Total Menopausal Seizure Assessments}}$$

8.6.2 Optimizing Medication Management During Menopause

Optimizing medication management during menopause is crucial. The Menopausal Medication Management Efficiency Quotient is calculated as:

$$\text{Menopausal Medication Management Efficiency Quotient} = \frac{\text{Optimized Drug Management Instances}}{\text{Total Menopausal Drug Management Cases}}$$

8.6.3 Managing Menopausal Symptoms and Seizure Risk

Managing menopausal symptoms to reduce seizure risk is practical. The Symptom Management and Seizure Prevention Quotient is expressed as:

$$\text{Symptom Management and Seizure Prevention Quotient}$$
$$= \frac{\text{Prevented Seizures Instances}}{\text{Total Menopausal Symptom Management Strategies Applied}}$$

8.6.4 Addressing Cognitive Changes and Memory Function

Addressing cognitive changes and memory function during menopause is crucial. The Cognitive Function and Memory Support Index is calculated as:

$$\text{Cognitive Function and Memory Support Index} = \frac{\text{Improved Cognitive Function Instances}}{\text{Total Menopausal Cognitive Support Interactions}}$$

8.6.5 Ensuring Emotional Well-being During Menopause

Ensuring emotional well-being during menopause is practical. The Menopausal Emotional Well-being Assurance Quotient is expressed as:

$$\text{Menopausal Emotional Well-being Assurance Quotient} = \frac{\text{Improved Well-being Instances}}{\text{Total Emotional Support Interactions}}$$

Efficiently navigating menopause and epilepsy involves optimizing these practical measures for a healthy and successful transition.

8.7 Reproductive Health and Epilepsy

Quickly understanding reproductive health and epilepsy is crucial. Let's explore this in a fast and practical manner.

8.7.1 Impact of Seizures on Reproductive Health

Understanding the impact of seizures on reproductive health is practical. The Seizure Impact on Reproductive Health Index is expressed as:

$$\text{Seizure Impact on Reproductive Health Index} = \frac{\text{Reproductive Health Compromised Instances}}{\text{Total Seizure Impact Assessments}}$$

8.7.2 Optimizing Medication Management for Fertility

Optimizing medication management for fertility is crucial. The Fertility Medication Management Efficiency Quotient is calculated as:

$$\text{Fertility Medication Management Efficiency Quotient} = \frac{\text{Optimized Drug Management Instances}}{\text{Total Fertility Drug Management Cases}}$$

8.7.3 Managing Seizures During Conception and Pregnancy

Managing seizures during conception and pregnancy is practical. The Conception and Pregnancy Seizure Management Quotient is expressed as:

$$\text{Conception and Pregnancy Seizure Management Quotient}$$
$$= \frac{\text{Managed Seizures Instances}}{\text{Total Conception and Pregnancy Seizure Management Strategies Applied}}$$

8.7.4   Addressing Hormonal Imbalance and Menstrual Cycle

Addressing hormonal imbalance and menstrual cycle irregularities is crucial. The Hormonal Balance and Menstrual Cycle Support Index is calculated as:

$$\text{Hormonal Balance and Menstrual Cycle Support Index} = \frac{\text{Improved Hormonal Balance Instances}}{\text{Total Reproductive Health Support Interactions}}$$

8.7.5   Ensuring Emotional Well-being in Reproductive Health

Ensuring emotional well-being in reproductive health is practical. The Reproductive Health Emotional Well-being Assurance Quotient is expressed as:

$$\text{Reproductive Health Emotional Well-being Assurance Quotient} = \frac{\text{Improved Well-being Instances}}{\text{Total Emotional Support Interactions}}$$

Efficiently managing reproductive health and epilepsy involves optimizing these practical measures for a healthy and successful journey to conception and beyond.

Chapter 9

Employment and Legal Considerations

9.1 Navigating Employment with Epilepsy

Quickly understanding how to navigate employment with epilepsy is crucial. Let's explore this in a fast and practical manner.

9.1.1 Disclosing Epilepsy to Employers

Deciding when and how to disclose epilepsy to employers is practical. The Epilepsy Disclosure Decision Quotient is expressed as:

$$\text{Epilepsy Disclosure Decision Quotient} = \frac{\text{Positive Disclosure Outcomes}}{\text{Total Disclosure Instances}}$$

9.1.2 Workplace Accommodations and Productivity

Negotiating workplace accommodations for increased productivity is crucial. The Accommodation Effectiveness Index is calculated as:

$$\text{Accommodation Effectiveness Index} = \frac{\text{Improved Productivity Instances}}{\text{Total Accommodation Requests}}$$

9.1.3 Managing Stress and Seizure Risk at Work

Managing stress to reduce seizure risk at work is practical. The Workplace Stress Management and Seizure Prevention Quotient is expressed as:

$$\text{Workplace Stress Management and Seizure Prevention Quotient}$$
$$= \frac{\text{Prevented Seizures Instances}}{\text{Total Workplace Stress Management Strategies Applied}}$$

9.1.4 Understanding Legal Rights and Protections

Understanding legal rights and protections in the workplace is crucial. The Legal Rights Awareness Quotient is calculated as:

$$\text{Legal Rights Awareness Quotient} = \frac{\text{Correctly Applied Legal Protections Instances}}{\text{Total Legal Consultations}}$$

9.1.5 Balancing Work and Health Considerations

Balancing work and health considerations is practical. The Work and Health Balance Quotient is expressed as:

$$\text{Work and Health Balance Quotient} = \frac{\text{Successfully Balanced Instances}}{\text{Total Work and Health Balancing Strategies Applied}}$$

Efficiently navigating employment with epilepsy involves optimizing these practical measures for a successful and fulfilling career.

9.2 Disclosing Your Condition at Work

Quickly understanding how to disclose your condition at work is crucial. Let's explore this in a fast and practical manner.

9.2.1 Choosing the Right Time to Disclose

Choosing the right time to disclose your condition is practical. The Disclosure Timing Decision Quotient is expressed as:

$$\text{Disclosure Timing Decision Quotient} = \frac{\text{Positive Timing Outcomes}}{\text{Total Disclosure Instances}}$$

9.2.2 Navigating Conversations with Supervisors

Navigating conversations with supervisors about your condition is crucial. The Supervisor Communication Effectiveness Index is calculated as:

$$\text{Supervisor Communication Effectiveness Index} = \frac{\text{Effective Communication Instances}}{\text{Total Supervisor Conversations}}$$

9.2.3 Requesting and Implementing Workplace Accommodations

Requesting and implementing workplace accommodations is practical. The Accommodation Request and Implementation Efficiency Quotient is expressed as:

$$\text{Accommodation Request and Implementation Efficiency Quotient}$$
$$= \frac{\text{Successfully Implemented Accommodations Instances}}{\text{Total Accommodation Requests}}$$

9.2.4 Minimizing Impact on Work Productivity

Minimizing the impact on work productivity is crucial. The Productivity Impact Mitigation Index is calculated as:

$$\text{Productivity Impact Mitigation Index} = \frac{\text{Mitigated Productivity Impact Instances}}{\text{Total Work Productivity Impact Occurrences}}$$

9.2.5 Understanding Legal Protections and Rights

Understanding legal protections and rights is practical. The Legal Protections Awareness Quotient is expressed as:

$$\text{Legal Protections Awareness Quotient} = \frac{\text{Correctly Applied Legal Protections Instances}}{\text{Total Legal Consultations}}$$

Efficiently disclosing your condition at work involves optimizing these practical measures for a successful and supportive workplace.

9.3   Legal Rights and Protections

Quickly understanding your legal rights and protections is crucial. Let's explore this in a fast and practical manner.

9.3.1   Knowing Your Rights in the Workplace

Knowing your rights in the workplace is practical. The Workplace Rights Awareness Quotient is expressed as:

$$\text{Workplace Rights Awareness Quotient} = \frac{\text{Correctly Applied Workplace Rights Instances}}{\text{Total Legal Consultations}}$$

9.3.2   Anti-Discrimination Laws and Compliance

Understanding anti-discrimination laws and ensuring compliance is crucial. The Anti-Discrimination Compliance Index is calculated as:

$$\text{Anti-Discrimination Compliance Index} = \frac{\text{Successfully Complied Instances}}{\text{Total Anti-Discrimination Compliance Checks}}$$

9.3.3   Navigating Reasonable Accommodations

Navigating reasonable accommodations within legal frameworks is practical. The Reasonable Accommodation Legal Navigation Quotient is expressed as:

$$\text{Reasonable Accommodation Legal Navigation Quotient}$$
$$= \frac{\text{Successfully Navigated Accommodations Instances}}{\text{Total Legal Navigation for Accommodations}}$$

9.3.4   Dealing with Workplace Harassment

Dealing with workplace harassment legally is crucial. The Workplace Harassment Legal Resolution Quotient is calculated as:

$$\text{Workplace Harassment Legal Resolution Quotient} = \frac{\text{Resolved Harassment Instances}}{\text{Total Harassment Legal Cases}}$$

9.3.5 Understanding Employment Contractual Rights

Understanding contractual rights in employment is practical. The Contractual Rights Awareness Quotient is expressed as:

$$\text{Contractual Rights Awareness Quotient} = \frac{\text{Correctly Applied Contractual Rights Instances}}{\text{Total Legal Consultations}}$$

Efficiently understanding legal rights and protections involves optimizing these practical measures for a secure and fair employment experience.

9.4 Reasonable Accommodations

Quickly understanding and navigating reasonable accommodations is crucial. Let's explore this in a fast and practical manner.

9.4.1 Identifying the Need for Accommodations

Identifying the need for accommodations is practical. The Accommodation Need Identification Quotient is expressed as:

$$\text{Accommodation Need Identification Quotient} = \frac{\text{Correctly Identified Accommodation Needs Instances}}{\text{Total Accommodation Assessments}}$$

9.4.2 Communicating Accommodation Requests

Communicating accommodation requests effectively is crucial. The Request Communication Effectiveness Index is calculated as:

$$\text{Request Communication Effectiveness Index} = \frac{\text{Effectively Communicated Requests Instances}}{\text{Total Accommodation Requests}}$$

9.4.3 Negotiating Accommodations with Employers

Negotiating accommodations with employers is practical. The Negotiation Success Quotient is expressed as:

$$\text{Negotiation Success Quotient} = \frac{\text{Successfully Negotiated Accommodations Instances}}{\text{Total Negotiation Attempts}}$$

9.4.4 Implementing and Assessing Accommodations

Implementing and assessing accommodations is crucial. The Accommodation Implementation and Effectiveness Quotient is calculated as:

$$\text{Accommodation Implementation and Effectiveness Quotient}$$
$$= \frac{\text{Successfully Implemented and Effective Accommodations Instances}}{\text{Total Accommodations Implemented}}$$

9.4.5 Legal Rights and Protections for Accommodations

Understanding legal rights and protections for accommodations is practical. The Legal Rights Awareness for Accommodations Quotient is expressed as:

$$\text{Legal Rights Awareness for Accommodations Quotient}$$
$$= \frac{\text{Correctly Applied Legal Protections for Accommodations Instances}}{\text{Total Legal Consultations for Accommodations}}$$

Efficiently navigating reasonable accommodations involves optimizing these practical measures for a workplace that supports your needs.

9.5 Insurance and Epilepsy

Quickly understanding insurance considerations related to epilepsy is crucial. Let's explore this in a fast and practical manner.

9.5.1 Navigating Health Insurance Policies

Navigating health insurance policies is practical. The Health Insurance Navigation Quotient is expressed as:

$$\text{Health Insurance Navigation Quotient} = \frac{\text{Successfully Navigated Policies Instances}}{\text{Total Health Insurance Navigation Attempts}}$$

9.5.2 Understanding Coverage for Epilepsy Medications

Understanding coverage for epilepsy medications is crucial. The Medication Coverage Awareness Quotient is calculated as:

$$\text{Medication Coverage Awareness Quotient} = \frac{\text{Correctly Applied Medication Coverage Instances}}{\text{Total Medication Coverage Inquiries}}$$

9.5.3 Exploring Disability Insurance Options

Exploring disability insurance options is practical. The Disability Insurance Exploration Quotient is expressed as:

$$\text{Disability Insurance Exploration Quotient}$$
$$= \frac{\text{Successfully Explored Disability Insurance Options Instances}}{\text{Total Disability Insurance Explorations}}$$

9.5.4 Understanding Workplace Disability Benefits

Understanding workplace disability benefits is crucial. The Workplace Disability Benefits Awareness Quotient is calculated as:

$$\text{Workplace Disability Benefits Awareness Quotient} = \frac{\text{Correctly Applied Workplace Disability Benefits Instances}}{\text{Total Workplace Disability Benefits Inquiries}}$$

9.5.5 Navigating Legal Protections for Insurance

Navigating legal protections related to insurance is practical. The Legal Protections Navigation Quotient is expressed as:

$$\text{Legal Protections Navigation Quotient} = \frac{\text{Successfully Navigated Legal Protections Instances}}{\text{Total Legal Protections Navigation Attempts}}$$

Efficiently understanding insurance considerations involves optimizing these practical measures for comprehensive coverage in managing epilepsy.

9.6   Disability Benefits

Quickly understanding disability benefits related to epilepsy is crucial. Let's explore this in a fast and practical manner.

9.6.1   Identifying Eligibility for Disability Benefits

Identifying eligibility for disability benefits is practical. The Eligibility Identification Quotient is expressed as:

$$\text{Eligibility Identification Quotient} = \frac{\text{Correctly Identified Eligibility Instances}}{\text{Total Eligibility Assessments}}$$

9.6.2   Navigating the Application Process

Navigating the disability benefits application process is crucial. The Application Navigation Quotient is calculated as:

$$\text{Application Navigation Quotient} = \frac{\text{Successfully Navigated Applications Instances}}{\text{Total Applications Submitted}}$$

9.6.3   Understanding the Approval Criteria

Understanding the approval criteria for disability benefits is practical. The Approval Criteria Awareness Quotient is expressed as:

$$\text{Approval Criteria Awareness Quotient} = \frac{\text{Correctly Applied Approval Criteria Instances}}{\text{Total Approval Criteria Inquiries}}$$

9.6.4   Dealing with Denials and Appeals

Dealing with denials and appeals for disability benefits is crucial. The Denials and Appeals Resolution Quotient is calculated as:

$$\text{Denials and Appeals Resolution Quotient} = \frac{\text{Successfully Resolved Denials and Appeals Instances}}{\text{Total Denials and Appeals Cases}}$$

9.6.5   Exploring Supplemental Security Income (SSI)

Exploring Supplemental Security Income (SSI) is practical. The SSI Exploration Quotient is expressed as:

$$\text{SSI Exploration Quotient} = \frac{\text{Successfully Explored SSI Instances}}{\text{Total SSI Explorations}}$$

Efficiently understanding disability benefits involves optimizing these practical measures for comprehensive support in managing epilepsy.

9.7   Planning for the Future

Quickly planning for the future related to employment and legal considerations is crucial. Let's explore this in a fast and practical manner.

9.7.1   Creating a Financial Plan

Creating a financial plan for the future is practical. The Financial Planning Effectiveness Quotient is expressed as:

$$\text{Financial Planning Effectiveness Quotient} = \frac{\text{Successfully Implemented Financial Plans Instances}}{\text{Total Financial Plans Created}}$$

9.7.2   Establishing an Emergency Fund

Establishing an emergency fund is crucial. The Emergency Fund Establishment Quotient is calculated as:

$$\text{Emergency Fund Establishment Quotient} = \frac{\text{Successfully Established Emergency Funds Instances}}{\text{Total Emergency Fund Setups}}$$

9.7.3   Exploring Retirement Savings Options

Exploring retirement savings options is practical. The Retirement Savings Exploration Quotient is expressed as:

$$\text{Retirement Savings Exploration Quotient} = \frac{\text{Successfully Explored Retirement Savings Instances}}{\text{Total Retirement Savings Explorations}}$$

9.7.4 Understanding Estate Planning

Understanding estate planning is crucial. The Estate Planning Awareness Quotient is calculated as:

$$\text{Estate Planning Awareness Quotient} = \frac{\text{Correctly Applied Estate Planning Instances}}{\text{Total Estate Planning Inquiries}}$$

9.7.5 Navigating Legal Documents

Navigating legal documents for future planning is practical. The Legal Documents Navigation Quotient is expressed as:

$$\text{Legal Documents Navigation Quotient} = \frac{\text{Successfully Navigated Legal Documents Instances}}{\text{Total Legal Document Navigations}}$$

Efficiently planning for the future involves optimizing these practical measures for a secure and well-prepared life with epilepsy.

Chapter 10

Technology and Epilepsy Management

10.1 Wearable Devices and Monitoring

Quickly understanding the role of wearable devices in epilepsy management is crucial. Let's explore this in a fast and practical manner.

10.1.1 Choosing the Right Wearable Device

Choosing the right wearable device is practical. The Wearable Device Selection Quotient is expressed as:

$$\text{Wearable Device Selection Quotient} = \frac{\text{Correctly Chosen Wearable Devices Instances}}{\text{Total Wearable Device Selections}}$$

10.1.2 Utilizing Monitoring Features

Utilizing monitoring features effectively is crucial. The Monitoring Features Utilization Quotient is calculated as:

$$\text{Monitoring Features Utilization Quotient} = \frac{\text{Successfully Used Monitoring Features Instances}}{\text{Total Monitoring Feature Utilizations}}$$

10.1.3 Interpreting Data and Reports

Interpreting data and reports from wearable devices is practical. The Data Interpretation Quotient is expressed as:

$$\text{Data Interpretation Quotient} = \frac{\text{Accurately Interpreted Data Instances}}{\text{Total Data Interpretations}}$$

10.1.4 Setting Up Alerts and Notifications

Setting up alerts and notifications is crucial. The Alerts and Notifications Setup Quotient is calculated as:

$$\text{Alerts and Notifications Setup Quotient} = \frac{\text{Successfully Configured Alerts Instances}}{\text{Total Alert Configurations}}$$

10.1.5 Integrating Wearable Data with Healthcare Providers

Integrating wearable data with healthcare providers is practical. The Data Integration Quotient is expressed as:

$$\text{Data Integration Quotient} = \frac{\text{Successfully Integrated Data Instances}}{\text{Total Data Integrations}}$$

Efficiently using wearable devices involves optimizing these practical measures for comprehensive epilepsy management.

10.2 Mobile Applications for Seizure Tracking

Quickly understanding the role of mobile applications in seizure tracking is crucial. Let's explore this in a fast and practical manner.

10.2.1 Choosing the Right Seizure Tracking App

Choosing the right seizure tracking app is practical. The App Selection Quotient is expressed as:

$$\text{App Selection Quotient} = \frac{\text{Correctly Chosen Apps Instances}}{\text{Total App Selections}}$$

10.2.2 Utilizing Seizure Logging Features

Utilizing seizure logging features effectively is crucial. The Seizure Logging Quotient is calculated as:

$$\text{Seizure Logging Quotient} = \frac{\text{Successfully Used Seizure Logging Instances}}{\text{Total Seizure Logging Sessions}}$$

10.2.3 Analyzing Seizure Trends

Analyzing seizure trends from mobile applications is practical. The Seizure Trends Analysis Quotient is expressed as:

$$\text{Seizure Trends Analysis Quotient} = \frac{\text{Accurately Analyzed Seizure Trends Instances}}{\text{Total Seizure Trends Analyses}}$$

10.2.4 Setting Up Medication Reminders

Setting up medication reminders is crucial. The Medication Reminder Setup Quotient is calculated as:

$$\text{Medication Reminder Setup Quotient} = \frac{\text{Successfully Configured Medication Reminders Instances}}{\text{Total Medication Reminder Configurations}}$$

10.2.5 Integrating App Data with Healthcare Providers

Integrating app data with healthcare providers is practical. The Data Integration Quotient is expressed as:

$$\text{Data Integration Quotient} = \frac{\text{Successfully Integrated Data Instances}}{\text{Total Data Integrations}}$$

Efficiently using mobile applications involves optimizing these practical measures for comprehensive seizure tracking in epilepsy management.

10.3 Telemedicine and Remote Consultations

Quickly understanding the role of telemedicine and remote consultations in epilepsy management is crucial. Let's explore this in a fast and practical manner.

10.3.1 Choosing the Right Telemedicine Platform

Choosing the right telemedicine platform is practical. The Platform Selection Quotient is expressed as:

$$\text{Platform Selection Quotient} = \frac{\text{Correctly Chosen Platforms Instances}}{\text{Total Platform Selections}}$$

10.3.2 Scheduling and Conducting Remote Consultations

Scheduling and conducting remote consultations effectively is crucial. The Remote Consultations Quotient is calculated as:

$$\text{Remote Consultations Quotient} = \frac{\text{Successfully Conducted Remote Consultations Instances}}{\text{Total Remote Consultations}}$$

10.3.3 Ensuring Patient Privacy and Data Security

Ensuring patient privacy and data security during telemedicine is practical. The Security Quotient is expressed as:

$$\text{Security Quotient} = \frac{\text{Maintained Patient Privacy Instances}}{\text{Total Security Checks}}$$

10.3.4 Utilizing Telemedicine for Medication Adjustments

Utilizing telemedicine for medication adjustments is crucial. The Medication Adjustment Quotient is calculated as:

$$\text{Medication Adjustment Quotient} = \frac{\text{Successfully Adjusted Medications Instances}}{\text{Total Medication Adjustments}}$$

10.3.5 Integrating Telemedicine Data with Healthcare Providers

Integrating telemedicine data with healthcare providers is practical. The Data Integration Quotient is expressed as:

$$\text{Data Integration Quotient} = \frac{\text{Successfully Integrated Data Instances}}{\text{Total Data Integrations}}$$

Efficiently using telemedicine involves optimizing these practical measures for comprehensive epilepsy management.

10.4 Emergency Alert Systems

Quickly understanding the role of emergency alert systems in epilepsy management is crucial. Let's explore this in a fast and practical manner.

10.4.1 Choosing the Right Emergency Alert System

Choosing the right emergency alert system is practical. The Alert System Selection Quotient is expressed as:

$$\text{Alert System Selection Quotient} = \frac{\text{Correctly Chosen Alert Systems Instances}}{\text{Total Alert System Selections}}$$

10.4.2 Configuring Emergency Contacts

Configuring emergency contacts effectively is crucial. The Emergency Contacts Configuration Quotient is calculated as:

$$\text{Emergency Contacts Configuration Quotient} = \frac{\text{Successfully Configured Emergency Contacts Instances}}{\text{Total Emergency Contacts Configurations}}$$

10.4.3 Testing Alert Systems

Testing alert systems is practical. The Alert System Testing Quotient is expressed as:

$$\text{Alert System Testing Quotient} = \frac{\text{Successfully Tested Alert Systems Instances}}{\text{Total Alert System Tests}}$$

10.4.4 Understanding Activation Protocols

Understanding activation protocols for emergency alert systems is crucial. The Activation Protocols Understanding Quotient is calculated as:

$$\text{Activation Protocols Understanding Quotient} = \frac{\text{Correctly Understood Activation Protocols Instances}}{\text{Total Activation Protocols Understandings}}$$

10.4.5   Integrating Alert System Data with Healthcare Providers

Integrating alert system data with healthcare providers is practical. The Data Integration Quotient is expressed as:

$$\text{Data Integration Quotient} = \frac{\text{Successfully Integrated Data Instances}}{\text{Total Data Integrations}}$$

Efficiently using emergency alert systems involves optimizing these practical measures for comprehensive epilepsy management.

10.5   Smart Home Technologies

Quickly understanding the role of smart home technologies in epilepsy management is crucial. Let's explore this in a fast and practical manner.

10.5.1   Choosing the Right Smart Home Devices

Choosing the right smart home devices is practical. The Device Selection Quotient is expressed as:

$$\text{Device Selection Quotient} = \frac{\text{Correctly Chosen Device Instances}}{\text{Total Device Selections}}$$

10.5.2   Setting Up Smart Home Monitoring

Setting up smart home monitoring is crucial. The Monitoring Setup Quotient is calculated as:

$$\text{Monitoring Setup Quotient} = \frac{\text{Successfully Set Up Monitoring Instances}}{\text{Total Monitoring Setups}}$$

10.5.3   Automating Seizure Detection

Automating seizure detection through smart home technologies is practical. The Seizure Detection Automation Quotient is expressed as:

$$\text{Seizure Detection Automation Quotient} = \frac{\text{Successfully Automated Seizure Detection Instances}}{\text{Total Seizure Detection Automations}}$$

10.5.4 Integrating Smart Home Data with Healthcare Providers

Integrating smart home data with healthcare providers is practical. The Data Integration Quotient is calculated as:

$$\text{Data Integration Quotient} = \frac{\text{Successfully Integrated Data Instances}}{\text{Total Data Integrations}}$$

Efficiently using smart home technologies involves optimizing these practical measures for comprehensive epilepsy management.

10.6 Assistive Devices

Quickly understanding the role of assistive devices in epilepsy management is crucial. Let's explore this in a fast and practical manner.

10.6.1 Choosing the Right Assistive Devices

Choosing the right assistive devices is practical. The Device Selection Quotient is expressed as:

$$\text{Device Selection Quotient} = \frac{\text{Correctly Chosen Device Instances}}{\text{Total Device Selections}}$$

10.6.2 Customizing Assistive Devices for Individual Needs

Customizing assistive devices for individual needs is crucial. The Customization Quotient is calculated as:

$$\text{Customization Quotient} = \frac{\text{Successfully Customized Devices Instances}}{\text{Total Customization Instances}}$$

10.6.3 Utilizing Wearable Assistive Technologies

Utilizing wearable assistive technologies is practical. The Wearable Technology Utilization Quotient is expressed as:

$$\text{Wearable Technology Utilization Quotient} = \frac{\text{Successfully Used Wearable Technologies Instances}}{\text{Total Wearable Technology Uses}}$$

10.6.4 Integrating Assistive Device Data with Healthcare Providers

Integrating assistive device data with healthcare providers is practical. The Data Integration Quotient is calculated as:

$$\text{Data Integration Quotient} = \frac{\text{Successfully Integrated Data Instances}}{\text{Total Data Integrations}}$$

Efficiently using assistive devices involves optimizing these practical measures for comprehensive epilepsy management.

10.7 Epilepsy and Social Media

Quickly understanding the role of social media in epilepsy management is crucial. Let's explore this in a fast and practical manner.

10.7.1 Leveraging Social Media for Support

Leveraging social media for support is practical. The Support Interaction Quotient is expressed as:

$$\text{Support Interaction Quotient} = \frac{\text{Positive Support Interactions}}{\text{Total Support Interactions}}$$

10.7.2 Educational Resources on Social Media

Utilizing educational resources on social media is crucial. The Education Access Quotient is calculated as:

$$\text{Education Access Quotient} = \frac{\text{Successfully Accessed Educational Resources}}{\text{Total Education Access Attempts}}$$

10.7.3 Connecting with Epilepsy Communities

Connecting with epilepsy communities on social media is practical. The Community Engagement Quotient is expressed as:

$$\text{Community Engagement Quotient} = \frac{\text{Engagement with Epilepsy Communities}}{\text{Total Engagement Attempts}}$$

10.7.4   Raising Awareness Through Social Media

Raising awareness through social media is practical. The Awareness Quotient is calculated as:

$$\text{Awareness Quotient} = \frac{\text{Successfully Raised Awareness Instances}}{\text{Total Awareness Attempts}}$$

Efficiently using social media involves optimizing these practical measures for comprehensive epilepsy management.

Chapter 11

Research and Advancements

11.1 Current Epilepsy Research

Quickly grasping the landscape of current epilepsy research is crucial. Let's explore this in a fast and practical manner.

11.1.1 Key Research Areas

Identifying key research areas helps navigate the vast field. The Research Focus Index is expressed as:

$$\text{Research Focus Index} = \frac{\text{Number of Key Research Areas Identified}}{\text{Total Research Areas Explored}}$$

11.1.2 Research Funding and Grants

Understanding research funding sources is vital. The Funding Success Quotient is calculated as:

$$\text{Funding Success Quotient} = \frac{\text{Successfully Secured Funding}}{\text{Total Funding Applications}}$$

11.1.3 Clinical Trial Awareness

Staying informed about ongoing clinical trials is practical. The Clinical Trial Awareness Score is expressed as:

$$\text{Clinical Trial Awareness Score} = \frac{\text{Awareness of Ongoing Clinical Trials}}{\text{Total Clinical Trials Monitored}}$$

11.1.4 Translating Research into Practice

Translating research into practical solutions is essential. The Translation Effectiveness Ratio is calculated as:

$$\text{Translation Effectiveness Ratio} = \frac{\text{Successful Translation Instances}}{\text{Total Translation Attempts}}$$

Efficiently navigating current epilepsy research involves optimizing these practical measures for advancements.

11.2 Clinical Trials and Participation

Understanding clinical trials is vital for staying updated on advancements. Let's explore this in a fast and practical manner.

11.2.1 Clinical Trial Basics

Getting acquainted with clinical trial fundamentals is essential. The Clinical Trial Fundamentals Score is expressed as:

$$\text{Clinical Trial Fundamentals Score} = \frac{\text{Understanding of Basic Clinical Trial Concepts}}{\text{Total Concepts Explored}}$$

11.2.2 Importance of Participation

Recognizing the importance of participant involvement is crucial. The Participation Significance Index is calculated as:

$$\text{Participation Significance Index} = \frac{\text{Acknowledgment of Participant Impact}}{\text{Total Perspectives Considered}}$$

11.2.3   Factors Influencing Participation

Identifying factors influencing participation is practical. The Participation Influencing Factors Matrix is expressed as:

$$\text{Participation Influencing Factors Matrix} = \begin{bmatrix} \text{Factor 1} & \text{Factor 2} & \dots & \text{Factor n} \\ \vdots & \vdots & \ddots & \vdots \\ \text{Factor m} & \text{Factor m+1} & \dots & \text{Factor m+n} \end{bmatrix}$$

11.2.4   Ethical Considerations

Understanding the ethical aspects of clinical trials is crucial. The Ethical Awareness Quotient is calculated as:

$$\text{Ethical Awareness Quotient} = \frac{\text{Awareness of Ethical Considerations}}{\text{Total Ethical Dimensions Explored}}$$

Efficiently navigating the realm of clinical trials involves optimizing these practical measures for research and advancements.

11.3   Emerging Therapies and Treatments

Navigating emerging therapies involves understanding the practical aspects. Let's delve into this in a quick and memorable way.

11.3.1   Therapeutic Landscape

Explore the evolving therapeutic landscape with the Therapeutic Horizon Map:

$$\text{Therapeutic Horizon Map} = \begin{bmatrix} \text{Current Therapies} & \text{Promising Candidates} \\ \text{Innovative Approaches} & \text{Cutting-edge Technologies} \end{bmatrix}$$

11.3.2   Innovative Technologies

Evaluate the impact of innovative technologies using the Technology Impact Index:

$$\text{Technology Impact Index} = \frac{\text{Technological Advancement Score}}{\text{Total Impact Dimensions}}$$

11.3.3   Promising Candidates

Identify promising candidates with the Candidate Potential Score:

$$\text{Candidate Potential Score} = \frac{\text{Effectiveness Index} \times \text{Safety Quotient}}{\text{Total Evaluation Criteria}}$$

11.3.4   Cutting-edge Research

Stay abreast of cutting-edge research with the Research Velocity Equation:

$$\text{Research Velocity} = \frac{\text{Discoveries per Month}}{\text{Total Research Dimensions}}$$

Embrace the dynamic world of emerging therapies by incorporating these practical measures for understanding and navigating advancements.

11.4   Genetic Research and Precision Medicine

Exploring genetic research and precision medicine in a fast and practical manner involves considering various aspects.

11.4.1   Understanding Genetic Research

Understanding the basics of genetic research is crucial. The Genetic Research Essentials Formula is expressed as:

$$\text{Genetic Research Essentials Formula} = \frac{\text{Understanding of Genetic Concepts}}{\text{Total Concepts Explored}}$$

11.4.2   Precision Medicine Fundamentals

Grasping the fundamentals of precision medicine is essential. The Precision Medicine Fundamentals Score is calculated as:

$$\text{Precision Medicine Fundamentals Score} = \frac{\text{Comprehension of Basic Precision Medicine Principles}}{\text{Total Principles Examined}}$$

11.4.3 Application of Genetic Findings

Applying genetic findings to precision medicine requires practical insights. The Application Proficiency Index is expressed as:

$$\text{Application Proficiency Index} = \frac{\text{Proficiency in Applying Genetic Insights}}{\text{Total Applications Considered}}$$

11.4.4 Molecular Insights in Precision Medicine

Understanding molecular aspects enhances precision medicine knowledge. The Molecular Insights Matrix is presented as:

$$\text{Molecular Insights Matrix} = \begin{bmatrix} \text{Insight 1} & \text{Insight 2} & \dots & \text{Insight n} \\ \vdots & \vdots & \ddots & \vdots \\ \text{Insight m} & \text{Insight m+1} & \dots & \text{Insight m+n} \end{bmatrix}$$

Efficiently navigating genetic research and precision medicine involves optimizing these practical measures for advancements.

11.5 Advancements in Imaging Technologies

Exploring the fast-paced world of advancements in imaging technologies requires a blend of real-world insights and practical knowledge.

11.5.1 Understanding Imaging Innovations

Understanding the basics of imaging innovations is critical. The Imaging Innovations Quotient is given by:

$$\text{Imaging Innovations Quotient} = \frac{\text{Understanding of Basic Imaging Concepts}}{\text{Total Concepts Explored}}$$

11.5.2 Practical Applications of Imaging

Applying imaging advancements practically is key. The Practical Application Score is calculated as:

$$\text{Practical Application Score} = \frac{\text{Application Proficiency in Imaging Technologies}}{\text{Total Applications Considered}}$$

11.5.3 Quantum Leap in Imaging

Embracing the quantum leap in imaging technologies involves recognizing key concepts. The Quantum Leap Index is expressed as:

$$\text{Quantum Leap Index} = \frac{\text{Recognition of Key Imaging Concepts}}{\text{Total Concepts in Quantum Leap}}$$

11.5.4 Chemical Insights in Imaging

Understanding the chemical aspects enhances imaging knowledge. The Chemical Insights Matrix is presented as:

$$\text{Chemical Insights Matrix} = \begin{bmatrix} \text{Insight 1} & \text{Insight 2} & \dots & \text{Insight n} \\ \vdots & \vdots & \ddots & \vdots \\ \text{Insight m} & \text{Insight m+1} & \dots & \text{Insight m+n} \end{bmatrix}$$

Efficiently navigating advancements in imaging technologies involves optimizing these practical measures for continuous progress.

11.6 Global Collaborations in Epilepsy Research

Dive into the dynamic realm of global collaborations in epilepsy research, where real-world impact meets practical insights.

11.6.1 Collaboration Effectiveness Index

Assessing the effectiveness of global collaborations requires a Collaboration Effectiveness Index, determined by:

$$\text{Collaboration Effectiveness Index} = \frac{\text{Number of Successful Collaborations}}{\text{Total Collaborations Attempted}}$$

11.6.2 Impact Factor of Collaborations

Quantifying the impact of collaborations is crucial. The Impact Factor is computed as:

$$\text{Impact Factor} = \frac{\text{Citations of Collaborative Research}}{\text{Total Citations in the Field}}$$

11.6.3 Mathematics of Collaboration

Expressing collaboration dynamics mathematically involves the Collaborative Equation:

$$\text{Collaborative Equation} : C = \frac{1}{\text{Distance}}$$

Here, C represents collaboration strength inversely proportional to distance.

11.6.4 Chemical Bonds in Global Collaboration

Analogous to chemical bonds, strong collaborations are formed. The Collaborative Bonds Formula is articulated as:

$$\text{Collaborative Bonds} = \frac{\text{Strength of Shared Goals}}{\text{Diversity in Collaborators}}$$

Navigating the world of global collaborations in epilepsy research requires a blend of strategic equations and collaborative chemistry.

11.7 Patient Advocacy and Involvement

Uncover the vital role of patients in shaping epilepsy research through active advocacy and involvement.

11.7.1 Patient Empowerment Index

Empowerment is quantified through the Patient Empowerment Index, calculated by:

$$\text{Patient Empowerment Index} = \frac{\text{Number of Advocacy Actions Taken}}{\text{Total Patient Population}}$$

11.7.2 Advocacy Impact Score

Assess the impact of patient advocacy with the Advocacy Impact Score, determined by:

$$\text{Advocacy Impact Score} = \frac{\text{Policy Changes Due to Advocacy}}{\text{Total Advocacy Efforts}}$$

11.7.3   Mathematics of Patient Involvement

Capture the mathematics of patient involvement through the Patient Engagement Equation:

$$\text{Patient Engagement Equation}: E = \frac{1}{\text{Distance from Patient Insights}}$$

Here, E signifies the strength of patient engagement inversely proportional to the distance from patient insights.

11.7.4   Chemistry of Patient Advocacy

Analogous to chemical reactions, patient advocacy involves forming impactful bonds. The Advocacy Bonds Formula is expressed as:

$$\text{Advocacy Bonds} = \frac{\text{Strength of Patient Voices}}{\text{Diversity in Advocacy Approaches}}$$

Navigate the landscape of epilepsy research advancements with the powerful blend of patient advocacy and mathematical insights.

Chapter 12

Epilepsy and Comorbidities

12.1 Understanding Comorbid Conditions

Delve into the intricate interplay between epilepsy and comorbidities through practical insights and mathematical perspectives.

12.1.1 Comorbidity Index

Quantify the impact of comorbidities with the Comorbidity Index, a mathematical representation:

$$\text{Comorbidity Index} = \frac{\text{Number of Comorbid Conditions}}{\text{Total Number of Patients}}$$

12.1.2 Risk Ratio Formula

Evaluate the risk of comorbidities using the Risk Ratio Formula:

$$\text{Risk Ratio} = \frac{\text{Probability of Comorbidity in Epileptic Patients}}{\text{Probability of Comorbidity in General Population}}$$

12.1.3 Intersection of Conditions

Visualize the overlap of epilepsy and comorbidities as a Venn diagram, where:

$$\text{Overlap} = \text{Number of Patients with Both Epilepsy and Comorbidity}$$

12.1.4 Mathematics of Treatment Strategies

Optimize treatment strategies using mathematical modeling:

$$\text{Optimal Treatment} = \frac{\text{Efficacy for Epilepsy} + \text{Efficacy for Comorbidity}}{\text{Total Treatment Burden}}$$

Navigate the complexities of epilepsy and comorbidities with a comprehensive blend of real-world insights and mathematical precision.

12.2 Managing Multiple Health Conditions

Unlock the practical strategies for navigating the complex terrain of epilepsy and comorbidities, blending real-world guidance with mathematical insights.

12.2.1 Holistic Treatment Approach

Adopt a holistic approach to treatment, where:

$$\text{Holistic Treatment Score} = \frac{\text{Effectiveness in Epilepsy} + \text{Effectiveness in Comorbidities}}{\text{Treatment Complexity}}$$

12.2.2 Health Optimization Equation

Maximize health outcomes with the Health Optimization Equation:

$$\text{Optimal Health} = \frac{\text{Epilepsy Control} \times \text{Comorbidity Management}}{\text{Treatment Burden}}$$

12.2.3 Strategies for Dual Management

Explore practical strategies for managing epilepsy and comorbidities simultaneously:

- Prioritize treatments with dual benefits.

- Optimize medication schedules to address both conditions.

- Leverage lifestyle modifications for holistic well-being.

12.2.4 Interactive Treatment Matrix

Visualize treatment interactions in a matrix, mapping the impact of each intervention on epilepsy and comorbidities.

	Epilepsy Control	Comorbidity Management	Treatment Burden
Treatment 1	+	+	−
Treatment 2	++	+	−−
Treatment 3	+	++	+

Embark on an integrative journey, optimizing the management of epilepsy and comorbidities with a synergy of practical wisdom and mathematical finesse.

12.3 Medication Interactions

Unravel the complexities of medication interactions in epilepsy and comorbidities, blending practical insights with mathematical precision.

12.3.1 Interactivity Quotient

Quantify the interactivity between medications using the Interactivity Quotient (IQ):

$$IQ = \frac{\text{Number of Medications} \times \text{Number of Potential Interactions}}{\text{Treatment Complexity}}$$

12.3.2 Optimizing Medication Regimens

Navigate medication interactions with these strategic maneuvers:

- **Smart Sequencing:** Order medications to minimize interactions.

- **Dose Balancing:** Adjust doses to optimize therapeutic effects.

- **Combination Compatibility:** Select combinations with synergistic benefits.

12.3.3 Interactive Medication Matrix

Visualize the medication landscape with an Interactive Medication Matrix:

	Epilepsy Medication 1	Epilepsy Medication 2	Comorbidity Medication
Effectiveness	++	+	+
Side Effects	−	− −	+
Interaction Potential	++	+	++

12.3.4 Mathematical Medication Harmony

Achieve mathematical harmony in medication management:

$$\text{Medication Harmony Index} =$$

$$\frac{\text{Effectiveness in Epilepsy} + \text{Effectiveness in Comorbidities} - \text{Interaction Potential}}{\text{Treatment Complexity}}$$

Embark on a journey of optimized medication management in epilepsy and comorbidities, where real-world pragmatism meets mathematical finesse.

12.4 Coordinating Care with Specialists

Embark on the journey of coordinating care with specialists in epilepsy and comorbidities, where practicality meets precision.

12.4.1 Collaborative Care Equation

Facilitate seamless collaboration among specialists with the Collaborative Care Equation:

$$\text{Collaborative Care Index} = \frac{\text{Number of Specialists}}{\text{Shared Treatment Modalities} + \text{Communication Frequency}}$$

12.4.2 Specialist Synchronization

Optimize care coordination by synchronizing specialists' efforts:

- **Treatment Overlaps:** Identify shared interventions to streamline care.

- **Communication Channels:** Establish efficient communication protocols.

- **Shared Decision Platforms:** Utilize platforms for unified treatment decisions.

12.4.3 Unified Care Plan

Craft a Unified Care Plan as the nucleus of coordinated care:

$$\text{Unified Care Plan} = \text{Epilepsy Treatment Plan} + \text{Comorbidity Management Plan} + \text{Integration Strategies}$$

12.4.4 Real-Time Intervention Matrix

Navigate care coordination dynamically with the Real-Time Intervention Matrix:

	Epileptologist	Neurologist	Comorbidity Specialist
Alert Triggers	Seizure Frequency	Neurological Changes	Comorbidity Exacerbation
Intervention Protocols	Medication Adjustments	Diagnostic Refinements	Comorbidity-specific Therapies
Communication Channels	Secure Messaging	Teleconferencing	Integrated Electronic Health Records

Table 12.1: Comparison of Specialists and Their Roles

Embark on a coordinated care odyssey, where specialists collaborate seamlessly, and patient outcomes take center stage.

12.5 Addressing Mental Health Comorbidities

Embark on a practical journey to address mental health comorbidities in epilepsy, where real-life solutions meet clinical insights.

12.5.1 Mental Health Integration Formula

Integrate mental health care seamlessly into epilepsy management with the Mental Health Integration Formula:

$$\text{Integration Index} = \frac{\text{Collaborative Interventions}}{\text{Communication Effectiveness} + \text{Patient Engagement}}$$

12.5.2 Patient-Centric Approach

Embrace a patient-centric approach in addressing mental health comorbidities:

- **Holistic Assessments:** Conduct comprehensive mental health assessments.

- **Shared Decision-Making:** Involve patients in treatment decisions.

- **Psychoeducation:** Equip patients with knowledge for self-management.

12.5.3 Therapeutic Synergy Protocol

Establish a Therapeutic Synergy Protocol for dual care:

$$\text{Synergy Index} = \frac{\text{Epilepsy Treatment Response}}{\text{Mental Health Stabilization}}$$

12.5.4 Crisis Management Algorithm

Navigate mental health crises with the Crisis Management Algorithm:

1. **Immediate Response:** Ensure patient safety.

2. **Communication Protocol:** Notify mental health and epilepsy specialists.

3. **Integrated Intervention:** Collaborate on a unified crisis intervention plan.

Empower patients to conquer mental health challenges alongside epilepsy, fostering a comprehensive path to well-being.

12.6 Nutritional Considerations with Comorbidities

Embark on a practical exploration of nutritional considerations in epilepsy, navigating the intersection of health and dietary choices.

12.6.1 Balanced Diet Equation

Maintain a balanced diet with the Balanced Diet Equation:

$$\text{Balanced Index} = \frac{\text{Nutrient Intake}}{\text{Caloric Needs}}$$

12.6.2 Seizure-Triggering Culprits

Identify and avoid potential seizure-triggering culprits:

- **Excitotoxins:** Minimize intake of MSG, aspartame, and excessive caffeine.

- **Sugar Stabilization:** Opt for low glycemic index foods to stabilize blood sugar.

- **Hydration Harmony:** Ensure adequate water intake for hydration balance.

12.6.3 Omega-3 Fatty Acid Synergy

Leverage Omega-3 Fatty Acid Synergy for brain health:

$$\text{Synergy Quotient} = \frac{\text{Eicosapentaenoic Acid (EPA)} + \text{Docosahexaenoic Acid (DHA)}}{\text{Omega-6 Fatty Acids}}$$

12.6.4 Micronutrient Optimization

Optimize micronutrient intake for holistic health:

$$\text{Optimization Score} = \frac{\text{Vitamins} + \text{Minerals}}{\text{Antioxidants}}$$

Navigate the nutritional landscape with precision, embracing a diet that harmonizes with epilepsy and comorbidities.

12.7 Balancing Treatment Approaches

Discover the art of balancing treatment approaches in managing epilepsy alongside comorbidities, combining pragmatism and mathematical precision.

12.7.1 Polytherapy Equation

Achieve optimal seizure control with the Polytherapy Equation:

$$\text{Polytherapy Index} = \frac{\text{Number of Medications}}{\text{Seizure Reduction}}$$

12.7.2   Lifestyle Integration

Incorporate lifestyle modifications seamlessly:

- **Activity Quotient (AQ):** Balance physical activity with rest for overall well-being.

- **Stress Resilience Score (SRS):** Gauge stress management effectiveness.

- **Sleep Optimization Index (SOI):** Enhance seizure control with sufficient and quality sleep.

12.7.3   Comorbidity Factor Analysis

Quantify the impact of comorbidities with the Comorbidity Factor:

$$\text{Comorbidity Factor} = \frac{\text{Comorbidity Severity}}{\text{Epilepsy Impact}}$$

Strike the right equilibrium, tailoring treatments to align with individualized needs for optimal outcomes.

Chapter 13

Community Outreach and Education

13.1 Raising Epilepsy Awareness

Ignite change through dynamic methods:

13.1.1 Awareness Propagation Formula

Utilize the Awareness Propagation Formula:

$$\text{Awareness} = \text{Initial Knowledge} + (\text{Effective Outreach} \times \text{Time})$$

13.1.2 Interactive Events

Organize impactful events:

- **Seizure Simulation Sessions:** Enhance understanding through immersive experiences.

- **Epilepsy Quotient (EQ) Quiz:** Gauge community knowledge and dispel myths.

13.1.3 Social Media Impact Score (SMIS)

Quantify online influence:

$$\text{SMIS} = \frac{\text{Engagement} + \text{Shares}}{\text{Followers}}$$

Empower communities with accurate information, breaking barriers and fostering empathy.

13.2   Community Education Programs

Elevate community understanding:

13.2.1   Knowledge Dissemination Rate (KDR)

$$\text{KDR} = \frac{\text{Information Shared}}{\text{Community Attendance}}$$

Implement engaging programs:

- **Epilepsy 101 Workshops:** Boost knowledge through interactive sessions.

- **Seizure Response Drills:** Equip communities with practical skills.

13.2.2   Interactive Learning Index (ILI)

Evaluate engagement:

$$\text{ILI} = \frac{\text{Interactive Tools Used}}{\text{Total Educational Tools}}$$

Maximize impact with tailored content, fostering a knowledgeable and supportive environment.

13.3   School and Workplace Education Initiatives

Empower the learning environment:

13.3.1   Impact Evaluation Score (IES)

Assess effectiveness:

$$\text{IES} = \frac{\text{Educational Impact}}{\text{Audience Size}}$$

Execute engaging initiatives:

- **School Awareness Programs:** Tailored sessions for students and teachers.

- **Workplace Inclusion Workshops:** Fostering understanding and support.

13.3.2 Participation Retention Ratio (PRR)

Measure retention:

$$\text{PRR} = \frac{\text{Participants Retained}}{\text{Initial Participants}}$$

Ensure lasting impact by adapting content to diverse learning environments.

13.4 Media and Epilepsy Representation

Shape narratives positively:

13.4.1 Media Perception Index (MPI)

Evaluate portrayal:

$$\text{MPI} = \frac{\text{Positive Mentions} - \text{Negative Mentions}}{\text{Total Mentions}}$$

Drive impactful initiatives:

- **Media Literacy Programs:** Equip communities to critically analyze portrayals.

- **Collaborate with Content Creators:** Encourage accurate representation in TV, movies, and online content.

13.4.2 Diversity Quotient (DQ)

Measure inclusivity:

$$\text{DQ} = \frac{\text{Representations of Epilepsy}}{\text{Total Representations}}$$

Advocate for diverse and authentic epilepsy stories in media platforms.

13.5 Volunteer Opportunities

Empower through active engagement:

13.5.1 Volunteer Impact Score (VIS)

Quantify contributions:

$$\text{VIS} = \frac{\text{Hours Volunteered} \times \text{Number of Engagements}}{\text{Positive Outcomes Achieved}}$$

Maximize impact:

- **Community Workshops:** Share expertise and support.

- **Online Mentorship Programs:** Connect volunteers with individuals seeking guidance.

13.5.2 Engagement Satisfaction Index (ESI)

Evaluate volunteer experience:

$$\text{ESI} = \frac{\text{Positive Experiences} - \text{Challenges Faced}}{\text{Total Experiences}}$$

Enhance programs based on feedback for a fulfilling volunteer experience.

13.6 Collaborating with Advocacy Organizations

Strengthen impact through partnerships:

13.6.1 Collaboration Success Index (CSI)

Evaluate collaboration effectiveness:

$$\text{CSI} = \frac{\text{Shared Goals Achieved} + \text{Effective Communication}}{\text{Challenges Faced}}$$

Maximize synergy:

- **Joint Events:** Combine resources for larger outreach.

- **Resource Sharing:** Optimize collective strengths for community benefit.

13.6.2 Advocacy Reach Potential (ARP)

Measure awareness dissemination:

$$ARP = \frac{\text{Collaborative Events} \times \text{Media Coverage}}{\text{Audience Reached}}$$

Amplify impact by reaching a wider audience through collaborative efforts.

13.7 Empowering Local Support Networks

Strengthening local bonds:

13.7.1 Community Cohesion Index (CCI)

Measure community strength:

$$CCI = \frac{\text{Active Participants} + \text{Shared Resources}}{\text{Challenges Faced}}$$

Promote collaboration:

- **Regular Meetings:** Foster face-to-face interactions.

- **Resource Pooling:** Combine local resources for impactful initiatives.

13.7.2 Empowerment Impact Quotient (EIQ)

Assess the effectiveness of empowerment initiatives:

$$EIQ = \frac{\text{Skill Development Programs} \times \text{Participation Rate}}{\text{Community Satisfaction}}$$

Empower through education and skill-building, ensuring active community involvement.

Chapter 14

Financial Considerations

14.1 Managing Medical Expenses

Navigate costs with precision:

14.1.1 Healthcare Budget Formula

Define your healthcare budget:

$$\text{Healthcare Budget} = \text{Income} - \text{Living Expenses} - \text{Emergency Fund}$$

Allocate a specific portion to medical needs.

14.1.2 Expense Coverage Ratio (ECR)

Assess medical expense coverage:

$$\text{ECR} = \frac{\text{Insurance Coverage}}{\text{Total Medical Expenses}}$$

Aim for a high ECR to minimize out-of-pocket expenses.

14.1.3 Medication Cost Efficiency Index (MCEI)

Evaluate medication expenses:

$$\text{MCEI} = \frac{\text{Therapeutic Effectiveness}}{\text{Medication Cost}}$$

Prioritize cost-effective treatments for better financial management.

14.2 Accessing Patient Assistance Programs

Unlock financial support:

14.2.1 Financial Needs Assessment

$$\text{Financial Need} = \text{Total Medical Expenses} - (\text{Insurance Coverage} + \text{Personal Budget})$$

Determine your financial gap for targeted assistance.

14.2.2 Patient Assistance Index (PAI)

$$\text{PAI} = \frac{\text{Financial Assistance Received}}{\text{Financial Need}}$$

Evaluate the effectiveness of assistance programs.

14.2.3 Medication Access Score (MAS)

$$\text{MAS} = \frac{\text{Medication Assistance Received}}{\text{Total Medication Cost}}$$

Optimize medication access with comprehensive assistance strategies.

14.3 Insurance Navigation

Sail through insurance complexities:

14.3.1 Out-of-Pocket Cost Estimation

$$\text{Out-of-Pocket Cost} = \text{Deductible} + \text{Co-insurance} + \text{Co-payment}$$

Calculate your potential financial responsibility.

14.3.2 Insurance Utilization Rate (IUR)

$$\text{IUR} = \frac{\text{Total Insurance Benefits Used}}{\text{Total Insurance Benefits Available}}$$

Maximize insurance coverage efficiently.

14.3.3 Appeal Success Rate (ASR)

$$\text{ASR} = \frac{\text{Successful Appeals}}{\text{Total Appeals Submitted}}$$

Enhance your appeal strategies for favorable outcomes.

14.4 Employment and Income Considerations

Navigate the financial landscape:

14.4.1 Net Income Calculation

$$\text{Net Income} = \text{Gross Income} - \text{Taxes}$$

Determine your actual income available for expenses.

14.4.2 Budgeting Formula

$$\text{Budget} = \text{Income} - \text{Expenses}$$

Develop a clear budget to manage your finances effectively.

14.4.3 Emergency Fund Target

$$\text{Emergency Fund Target} = \text{Monthly Expenses} \times \text{Number of Months}$$

Ensure financial security with a robust emergency fund.

14.5 Financial Planning with Chronic Illness

Strategize for financial well-being:

14.5.1   Savings Growth Calculation

$$\text{Future Value} = \text{Present Value} \times (1 + \text{Interest Rate})^{\text{Time}}$$

Estimate your savings' future value with compounded interest.

14.5.2   Debt Repayment Formula

$$\text{Monthly Payment} = \frac{\text{Loan Amount} \times \text{Interest Rate}}{1 - (1 + \text{Interest Rate})^{-\text{Number of Payments}}}$$

Plan your debt repayment with a structured monthly approach.

14.5.3   Risk Tolerance Assessment

Assess your risk tolerance to make informed investment decisions.

14.5.4   Investment Portfolio Diversification

$$\text{Portfolio Diversification} = \frac{\text{Investment in Asset A}}{\text{Total Portfolio Value}} \times 100$$

Diversify your investments to manage risk effectively.

14.6   Government Assistance Programs

Explore support options:

14.6.1   Eligibility Criteria

$$\text{Eligibility Score} = \frac{\text{Household Income}}{\text{Number of Dependents}}$$

Evaluate eligibility based on income and dependents.

14.6.2   Benefits Calculation

$$\text{Total Benefits} = \text{Benefit Rate} \times \text{Number of Eligible Months}$$

Calculate potential benefits by considering the benefit rate and eligibility duration.

14.6.3 Budgeting for Assistance

$$\text{Allocated Budget} = \frac{\text{Total Benefits}}{\text{Number of Months}}$$

Plan your budget effectively with the allocated assistance.

14.6.4 Government Aid Impact

$$\text{Income Change} = \text{New Income} - \text{Old Income}$$

Assess the impact of government aid on your overall income.

14.7 Legal Aid and Financial Advocacy

Navigate legal and financial support:

14.7.1 Legal Consultation

$$\text{Legal Consultation Score} = \frac{\text{Legal Issues}}{\text{Financial Resources}}$$

Evaluate the need for legal aid based on the severity of legal issues and available financial resources.

14.7.2 Financial Advocacy Impact

$$\text{Financial Impact} = \text{New Financial Status} - \text{Previous Financial Status}$$

Assess the impact of legal aid and financial advocacy on your overall financial status.

14.7.3 Negotiation Strategies

Implement effective negotiation strategies to improve financial outcomes.

14.7.4 Legal Protection Plan

$$\text{Legal Protection Score} = \frac{\text{Legal Safeguards}}{\text{Financial Risk}}$$

Determine the adequacy of legal safeguards in protecting against financial risks.

Chapter 15

Epilepsy and Aging

15.1   Understanding Aging and Epilepsy

Explore the dynamics of aging with epilepsy:

15.1.1   Epilepsy Incidence with Age

$$\text{Incidence Rate} = \frac{\text{Number of New Cases}}{\text{Total Population at Risk}} \times 100$$

Understand how the incidence of epilepsy changes with age.

15.1.2   Age-Related Risk Factors

Identify and manage age-specific risk factors contributing to epilepsy.

15.1.3   Cognitive Health Metrics

$$\text{Cognitive Health Index} = \frac{\text{Cognitive Performance}}{\text{Age-related Expectations}} \times 100$$

Evaluate cognitive health in relation to age-related expectations.

15.1.4   Medication Adjustments

Adjust epilepsy medications based on age-related physiological changes.

15.1.5 Lifestyle Modifications

Implement age-appropriate lifestyle changes for optimal epilepsy management.

15.1.6 Brain Health Exercises

Engage in brain health exercises to promote cognitive well-being.

15.2 Epilepsy in the Elderly

Uncover insights into epilepsy in the elderly:

15.2.1 Prevalence

$$\text{Prevalence} = \frac{\text{Number of Cases}}{\text{Total Elderly Population}} \times 100$$

Understand the prevalence of epilepsy in the elderly population.

15.2.2 Risk Factors

Identify and manage specific risk factors associated with epilepsy in older individuals.

15.2.3 Cognitive Challenges

Explore cognitive challenges and address them for improved quality of life.

15.2.4 Polypharmacy

Manage polypharmacy challenges, optimizing medication regimens for elderly patients.

15.2.5 Seizure Triggers

Identify and mitigate seizure triggers tailored to the elderly population.

15.2.6 Neuroprotective Measures

Implement neuroprotective measures to support brain health in the aging population.

15.2.7 Community Support

Foster community support systems for elderly individuals living with epilepsy.

15.3 Medication Adjustments in Aging

Navigate the intricacies of medication adjustments for elderly individuals with epilepsy:

15.3.1 Pharmacokinetic Changes

$$\text{Dose}_{\text{adjusted}} = \frac{\text{Dose}_{\text{original}}}{\text{Age Factor}}$$

Understand pharmacokinetic changes in the elderly and calculate adjusted medication doses.

15.3.2 Renal Function Assessment

Regularly assess renal function for accurate medication dosage adjustments.

15.3.3 Liver Function Monitoring

Monitor liver function to ensure optimal drug metabolism in aging individuals.

15.3.4 Polypharmacy Considerations

Manage polypharmacy challenges, balancing multiple medications for elderly patients.

15.3.5 Individualized Treatment Plans

Develop personalized treatment plans, considering comorbidities and overall health.

15.3.6 Adherence Strategies

Implement adherence strategies to support consistent medication intake in the elderly.

15.3.7 Regular Medication Reviews

Conduct regular reviews to adapt medications based on the evolving health of elderly patients.

15.4   Cognitive and Memory Concerns

Address cognitive and memory issues in aging individuals with epilepsy:

15.4.1   Neurocognitive Assessments

Conduct regular neurocognitive assessments to evaluate cognitive function.

15.4.2   Memory Enhancement Strategies

Implement memory enhancement strategies for individuals experiencing memory issues.

15.4.3   Cognitive Rehabilitation

Introduce cognitive rehabilitation programs to improve cognitive abilities.

15.4.4   Mental Stimulation Activities

Encourage mental stimulation activities to support cognitive health in elderly patients.

15.4.5   Lifestyle Modifications

Promote a healthy lifestyle with proper nutrition and regular physical exercise.

15.4.6   Medication Adjustments

Consider medication adjustments to minimize cognitive side effects in aging individuals.

15.4.7   Supportive Environment

Create a supportive environment for elderly individuals with epilepsy to enhance cognitive well-being.

15.5   Long-Term Care Planning

Address long-term care planning for elderly individuals with epilepsy:

15.5.1   Caregiver Support

Provide resources and support for caregivers of elderly individuals with epilepsy.

15.5.2 Healthcare Proxy

Establish a healthcare proxy to ensure medical decisions align with the patient's preferences.

15.5.3 Legal Documentation

Prepare legal documents, such as advance directives, to guide medical care decisions.

15.5.4 Financial Planning

Assist in financial planning for long-term care, considering medical expenses and support services.

15.5.5 Residential Options

Explore suitable residential options that cater to the specific needs of elderly individuals with epilepsy.

15.5.6 Community Resources

Connect with community resources that offer assistance and services for aging individuals with epilepsy.

15.5.7 Regular Health Check-ups

Schedule regular health check-ups to monitor and address the evolving healthcare needs of elderly patients.

15.6 Supporting Caregivers

Assist caregivers of elderly individuals with epilepsy:

15.6.1 Education and Training

Provide educational resources and training to equip caregivers with necessary skills in epilepsy management.

15.6.2 Respite Care Services

Offer respite care services to provide caregivers with periodic breaks to avoid burnout.

15.6.3 Emotional Support

Establish emotional support programs to address the mental health and well-being of caregivers.

15.6.4 Community Networks

Connect caregivers with community networks and support groups to share experiences and insights.

15.6.5 Medical Training

Provide basic medical training to caregivers for emergency situations and seizure response.

15.6.6 Financial Assistance

Explore financial assistance programs to alleviate the economic burden on caregivers.

15.6.7 Legal Guidance

Offer legal guidance to caregivers for issues related to healthcare decisions and support.

15.7 Maintaining Quality of Life

Strategies to maintain a high quality of life for elderly individuals with epilepsy:

15.7.1 Regular Exercise

Encourage regular physical activity to promote overall well-being and reduce seizure risk.

15.7.2 Healthy Diet

Advise a balanced and nutritious diet, considering potential interactions with anti-epileptic drugs.

15.7.3 Cognitive Stimulation

Engage in activities that stimulate the mind, such as puzzles or memory exercises.

15.7.4 Social Connections

Foster social interactions to prevent isolation and promote emotional health.

15.7.5 Medication Adherence

Ensure strict adherence to medication schedules to control seizures effectively.

15.7.6   Regular Medical Check-ups

Schedule routine medical check-ups to monitor overall health and address issues promptly.

15.7.7   Adequate Sleep

Promote healthy sleep habits as disrupted sleep patterns can trigger seizures.

15.7.8   Emergency Preparedness

Have an emergency plan in place to manage seizures effectively when they occur.